FALLING THROUGH THE CEILING
Our ADHD Family Memoir

Falling Through the Ceiling, Our ADHD Family Memoir © 2018 by Audrey R. Jones & Larry A. Jones, MD

First Edition

No part of this book may be reproduced in any written, electronic, recording, or photocopying form without written permission of the publisher. The exception would be in the case of brief quotations embodied in critical articles or reviews and pages where the publisher specifically grants permission.

Although every precaution has been taken to verify the accuracy of the information contained herein, the authors and publisher assume no responsibility for any errors or omissions. This publication is designed to provide accurate and authoritative information. It is sold with the understanding that the publisher is not engaged in providing psychological, legal, financial, or other professional services. If expert services or professional counseling is needed, the services of a competent professional shall be sought.

No liability is assumed for damages that may result from the use of information contained within.

Library of Congress Control Number: 2018904194

ISBN: 978-0-692-09988-9

Publisher: Enable Tables Media
Smart Management, Inc.
PO Box 23338
St. Louis, MO 63156

Website: enabletables.com
Printed in the United States

FALLING THROUGH THE CEILING
OUR ADHD FAMILY MEMOIR

Audrey R. Jones & Larry A. Jones, MD

To our parents, who gave us all they had.
To our sons, who endured all we gave them.
To our extended family, who loved us through the journey.

Acknowledgments

We are most thankful for our parents. Without Jackie and Willie Mae Robinson, who parented both of us with love and constant support through the early years of marriage and parenting, we probably would not have celebrated over 45 years of marriage. We continue to appreciate the love and sacrifices of Alberta Jones and Vernon Goward, the mother, grandmother team who gave Larry a "two parent" family

We are grateful to our friends and family who have helped to guide us and smooth out the wrinkles of living with the challenges of ADHD, especially those days when we thought things were out of control, and we were *falling through the ceiling*.

We especially appreciate the assistance of Jo Lena Johnson and Dolores B. Malcolm for your invaluable coaching and editing. Addressing the multiple facets of each son's ADHD required expertise, patience and support from a variety of educators, counselors and therapists. They were objective and empathetic with our sons and several even became long-term members of our village. We especially thank our personal therapists who encouraged us to document our lives so that other families would know that they are not alone.

When we attended the 2017 International Conference on ADHD: "Connect & Recharge" sponsored by CHADD and ADDA we learned so much from the training sessions led by the experts. However, it was the attendees who like Larry were also diagnosed with ADHD, and their spouses that also inspired us to share our stories as a way to encourage others to share theirs.

Contents

Forward 11

Introduction 13

Suffering in Silence 15

From Whence We Came 17

Audrey, Straight Out of Kansas 19

Larry Had One Shot 23

Our Impaired Courtship 29

Helicopter Over Hopkins 33

I'm Gonna Make it Happen! 37

Motherhood: Triple Blessings in the Midst of Distraction 39

Becoming a Dad 47

Fatherhood, Making It Happen 49

Lack of Self-Control and Impulsivity Are Key Traits of ADHD 53

Locking the Door 55

The Droopy Eye 59

I Know This Doesn't Sound Funny But 61

Present Yet Disconnected 63

Faking Seizures 65

Creativity and Hyperfocus 69

Teenager Alone in Paris 73

Impulsivity 75

Rob in Transition 77

Say What? ADHD? No, Not We! 81

The Many Faces of ADHD 85

The ADD/ADHD Iceberg	87
Nothing Is Normal	91
Building a Village for Our Sons	93
Build a Village of Educators and Others Who Support the Adolescent's Goals	97
He Didn't Remove the Pins	99
Samurai Swordsmen	103
The Jones Wrecking Crew	111
The Last Family Vacation	119
Sex	125
The Enable Table	135
Falling Through the Ceiling	141
Giving Our Sons a New Start	143
Being the Enabler Turns Deadly	147
ADHD Affects Everything from Money to Marriage	153
Money Matters and Materialism	155
Love, Friendship, and Marriage	161
Larry's Advice, Especially for Fathers	167
Audrey's Advice, Especially for Mothers	171
For Parents: Lessons from Our Lives	175
Final Thoughts	179
Frustration to Resilience	183
Appendix: What is ADHD?	185
Appendix: Advocating for Diagnosis and Treatment	187
Glossary of Terms	191
Resources	195
References	197

FOREWORD

Falling Through the Ceiling: Our ADHD Family Memoir, is a poignant book about the challenges encountered by both parents and children as they cope with attention deficit/hyperactivity disorder (ADHD). The authors, Audrey and Larry Jones, provide a sensitive, knowledgeable, and often humorous account of the obstacles inherent in raising children with ADHD. They describe their personal journey, from dating to marriage to parenthood and grandparenthood. Although they put their experience in the context of every family's aspirations, they also highlight the unique experiences of Black American families who are navigating the complex process of coming to terms with ADHD. The authors take the reader through the early childhood years, when ADHD can result in academic frustrations and often dramatic childhood pranks. They then move on through adolescence and young adulthood, when, for youth with ADHD, the launch into independence can be fraught with more than the average obstacles. As the authors tell their family's story, each of them stops along the way to reflect on the personal impact of the children's challenges and to share their perspective's on how they might have handled things differently. This book will be an inspiration for the thousands of families who are confronted with ADHD.

E. Walker

Elaine F. Walker, Ph.D.
Charles Howard Candler Professor of Psychology and Neuroscience
Director, Mental Health and Development Program
Emory University
Atlanta, GA 30322

INTRODUCTION

For us *Falling Through the Ceiling* is a blend of love, humor and real-life irony. We make sense of the nonsensical by shedding light on our challenges of living with attention deficit disorder (ADHD).

Our stories are examples of the things that can happen when ADHD runs rampant and untreated for parent and three sons. That is what defines the universality of our stories. We fell into the same trap as many other parents, thinking that Drew, Jay, and Rob were just lazy and willfully not completing assignments in school. Parenting is probably the most humbling experience of your life. Few of us are trained in parenting and we encounter events in our children's lives, which should lead us to professional counselors and therapists. Our darling children can throw us off kilter because they really do the darndest things.

We were struggling to make it and created codependency and unhealthy enabling habits. What we did, and what we didn't do, to help our sons didn't work, many times. The behaviors simply continued and morphed. If we had it to do all over again, we would have done things better and differently. Hopefully our stories will give other parents relief, support, courage and solutions.

Suffering in Silence

"Defiant, daring behavior leading to failures, including sexual acting out, running away from home and inviting danger, were our reality in our house full of ADHD." – Audrey and Larry, parents

We were an upwardly mobile, middle-class family. If you asked our friends, they would have said we were loving, active, hardworking and provided for our children. As our careers took off, we earned more income, moved to better neighborhoods, upgraded schools and cars, and we did the things most people want to do…we weren't trying to keep up, we *were* the "Jones family," after all.

Yet our friends and others didn't know what was happening on the inside. What happened in our house stayed in our house. Our house full of attention deficit hyperactive disorder (ADHD) was an open minefield of poor decision-making, risky choices, immature behavior as well as lyin' and denyin.' We had issues and covered them up by solving the problems, enabling the behavior and giving in to the bright ideas of the day.

Our sons were well-mannered, handsome and smart, yet our house was full of failure, impulse and self-focus, especially as our three boys aged. Nobody ever knew what was happening because we, the parents, got them out of trouble. As the years went by, more and more "below-the-surface" activities started emerging. These behaviors were not obvious to the naked eye but were present and intrusive, just like the unseen foreboding presence of an iceberg. Eighty percent of an iceberg is under water, massive and dangerous, able to sink ships like the *Titanic*. This is how attention deficit hyperactivity disorder (ADHD) can affect families, especially when undiagnosed or ignored.

Without humor and hope, we would not have made it. If our stories resonate with your family experiences, perhaps we have something in common.

From Whence We Came

Before we introduce our family, it's important to set the stage from whence we came. We want you and anyone who reads our stories to have hope, determination and perseverance to fight for your dreams.

Every decision we made was to give our sons better and more than we had. Right or wrong, good or bad, we did our best, flailing along the way. We stayed together, and here we are.

Audrey, Straight Out of Kansas

"My parents met and married late in life, not planning to have children. They were both over 40, after all." – Audrey

My father had been married before, and from that union came two sons and a daughter. During childbirth, his wife passed as she was delivering my half-sister, Charity. My father and Charity didn't have a close relationship. She was raised by his sister, a single aunt who was childless. He took care of her throughout her life, however, he never had an active role in her upbringing. Unlike Charity, my brothers grew up with Dad in Kansas.

My mother had been pregnant once in her early 30s. She lost the baby when she fell down a flight of stairs shortly before her first husband died under mysterious circumstances while on a hunting trip.

My father thought he was sterile because he had chicken pox in his late 30s, a myth from that time, so they weren't worried about birth control. My mother began having hot flashes and went to the neighborhood general practitioner, who administered a dose of hormones. He inadvertently gave her a month's dosage at one time. That stimulated ovulation. At 43 years old, my mother found herself pregnant and I was born in the spring of 1950. Being "old parents," they were both determined to do their best by me, despite their past relationships and choices.

My dad always worked at least two jobs at a time. He never minded it because it allowed my mom to be a stay-at-home mother, plus he liked being busy, working. Not educated, he was self-taught and learned enough skills to work in manufacturing plants, manage parking garages and eventually becoming the maintenance manager for a union-owned office building. That position afforded us many benefits, which I didn't appreciate at the time. I just knew he wore a uniform and carried a lunch box. As a child, I thought he was a janitor. I didn't understand that he was a man of such dexterity. Managing that building, he did everything from fixing the furnace to assembling furniture to training and supervising others to do the same thing. He drove a taxi at night, and on Sundays, he drove the church bus and was a deacon, all at the same time!

Middle-Class Mindset and Values

My parents owned our modest home, and thanks to my dad's connections and ingenuity, we lived a middle-class life in the Black area of Kansas City, Kansas. Our community was self-sufficient and segregated at the same time. During those days, most Blacks lived on the north side, and our neighborhood was filled with doctors, lawyers, educators and all manner of blue-collar workers. Our family always managed to have updated cars, we took annual vacations, and we were extremely active in church and the "Black" YWCA branch.

In the spring of 1966, right after my 16th birthday, I became the first person in our little family to fly on a plane. To this day, I don't know how my parents managed to get me the opportunity, but my life would never be the same after that experience. Dressed in my Sunday best, my parents were so proud to see me board that TWA flight as a delegate to the National YWCA convention in Boston. Chaperoned by trusted members of our small African American community, I felt like Dorothy, getting the heck out of Kansas that day. Since I was so young, I had no appreciation of the sacrifices my parents had made to launch me into the world; I was just happy to be out. While on the trip, I learned of the number of colleges in the Boston and New England area.

I had to go back, and I did. In 1967, I am confident through prayer and asking everyone she knew, Mama found the Wellesley Club of Kansas City. In the midst of the civil rights movement, the Wellesley women helped their first Black Kansas City applicant to waive fees and have a local interview. With excellent grades and a decent SAT score, I, the first Black Woman from Kansas City, became a member of the 1968 freshman class at the prestigious women's college outside of Boston. For the next five years I actively recruited at least one Black woman to attend Wellesley each year.

Before leaving for Wellesley, my mother, over 60 years old at the time, armed me with two pieces of relationship advice. The first: "Get to know the man before you marry him." This was based on her own experience and regrets. She was extremely unhappy in her first marriage because she married innocently. He was her first, for everything, and because she was older when she did so, it was a bad experience for her. She didn't want me to repeat her mistake. Her marriage to my father was the total opposite, and she wanted me to have that type of joy and fulfillment. Second, she said, *"Don't marry a doctor or a preacher."* My mother's best friend was our local doctor's mistress, and she just felt that doctors had too much freedom, money, power and opportunity to be philanderers. She looked at preachers the same way. She didn't want me to be subjected to a either situation.

> "*I met Audrey at a party during my junior year on a road trip to Boston, 100 miles away. We heard there were 100 African American freshman girls at Wellesley. That was Saturday night, February 21, 1970. Meeting Audrey meant the end of my hyper focus, new adventures, more hard work and the beginning of an amazing courtship and subsequent marriage.*" – Larry

Larry Had One Shot

"I am a second-generation only child, thus I have no siblings and my mother had no siblings. I never knew my father. Being raised by my mother and grandmother meant many restrictions. As a result, I was a sheltered, single-focused adolescent." – Larry

I always knew I only had one shot. Growing up, we were poor, and I took things seriously because I had to. My life was complicated, sad and quite different from the life and opportunities we provided for our sons. I didn't know I had ADD until my youngest son, Rob, was in elementary school. People may wonder how I made it through Wesleyan, an elite New England college, medical school, and being a husband and a father given my undiagnosed condition. It goes back to the title of this chapter: I always knew I only had one shot because of my circumstances.

My mother and grandmother were my parents. I never knew my father. They never talked about him, even when I wanted to know who and where he was. When I was 11 or 12, I discovered a note he wrote on the inside of an armoire in my bedroom, which I used daily. It was as though one day the writing on the inside door suddenly became visible, though it had been there all my life. The note said he was leaving my mother, and it was signed Horace Jones. I never knew his name until that point. Seeing this note forced me to start asking new questions about him. I was told that he had moved away to Mansfield, Ohio. I'm sure my father left because of my grandmother—that he couldn't get my mother away from her. There is no way that any man with self-pride could have lived with my grandmother. I don't know if my parents married or not. By adulthood, I had no real desire to look for him because I felt he had no desire to look for me. *Why would I look for a man who abandoned me as a baby?*

In 2009, after our youngest son had relocated to Ohio, we were at a genealogy center using Ancestry.com, learning about my wife's family. Rob insisted that I look up mine, as he was hoping to find his grandfather and perhaps some long-lost uncles. It only took me 15 minutes to find the information. I learned my father had settled in Mansfield, had a couple of children and was deceased. I was surprised it was so easy. After that, I left it alone.

My mother became ill with cancer in 1965 when I was 15, the summer after my sophomore year in high school. My grandmother and I were devastated. We were poor and had no insurance. My mother's medical care was at the city clinic at the University of Tennessee Hospital. She had provided most of the family income, but with her illness and subsequent treatment, she was unable to return to work.

"What are we going to do?" We prayed for my mother to be healed, although the treatment made her sicker than she was before. My grandmother, Ninny, decided to quit her job as a domestic worker (maid) to care for my mother, noting her weakened condition after her radiation treatments. Now there was no family income. Ninny had faith that the Lord would provide for us. We continued to pray.

At that point, our church and neighborhood provided food, money and the support of their prayers. We never missed a meal, and I was able to continue school without interruption. Our landlord helped us by allowing us to delay paying the rent for several months until we could apply for welfare. I took care of the family chores, the washing, the grocery shopping as well as some of the cooking in addition to helping care for my ailing mother. One of the many rules I had was that I had to come straight home from school, with no extracurricular activities. As a result, I was a sheltered, lonely boy.

When my world started falling apart, I had no one to talk to about how I felt about my mother's illness. I was worried and aching to unload the burden of my mother's illness to a sympathetic ear. I asked the doctor caring for my mother if she would survive. He assured me that she would be okay, but I knew I was losing her. I tried to talk to my grandmother about my concerns, but she was in complete denial. I began to talk to three of my teachers about my mother's illness. They listened and supported me through this period. These guardian angels, along with prayer and faith, got me through. The village—my teachers, the church and our neighbors—blanketed us with their love and prayers.

My plan since age seven was to become a physician. *How was I going to go to college without any money and no family financial support?* I had faith that there would be a way when the time came. One of those three teachers was now my guidance counselor. She had been my mother's 12th-grade homeroom teacher. She made sure that I was picked for every summer program and opportunity to meet with college recruiters. She and the other two teachers helped me to get test fees and application fees waived, which gave me the opportunity to compete for national scholarships.

In the 1960s, children identified as gifted, though poor, were expected to become doctors, lawyers or teachers. Ms. Addie, my counselor, organized the faculty to make sure I got scholarships, transportation and entrance to Wesleyan University, my first choice. They put their support behind me, believing I was a child who could actually become a doctor. Thanks to their support, I was able to get back and forth to Connecticut.

College on the East Coast

In August before leaving for college, three Black Wesleyan students from Memphis met with me to set my expectations. Wesleyan was a strenuous academic environment. It was an all-male private school, and at the time, there were less than 15 Black men on campus. My freshman class entered with 35 Black men, the largest by far in the school's history. If I was going to complete the premed program there, I had to compete with young men from around the world. I had to jump in running in order to stay in the pack. I was hyperfocused on my one shot for those first two years.

Then I met the love of my life during my junior year, the year I transferred to the premed program at Johns Hopkins with automatic admission to the medical school. That last premed year went well, but the rigorous curriculum of the first year of medical school tested my every fiber. The difficulty of the studies, the isolation and my poor note-taking skills made it difficult to keep up. I began to fall asleep in class, believing that was happening because I found the lectures to be boring. The ongoing long-distance relationship with Audrey and working part-time in addition to my medical school studies resulted in poor performance on final exams that semester. I failed the first year of medical school. That was a big blow that shook me to my core. *How could I continue at Johns Hopkins when everybody would know I had failed that first year? What was I going to do? Transferring to another medical school was not an option. Was I going to give up my dream and quit? No!* It took my medical school advisor and my fiancé to shake me back to reality. I had to swallow my pride and start over. I prayed for the strength and fortitude to continue. That year of distraction had cost me, but I truly feel that I could not have finished without my greatest cheerleader, Audrey. She became my support and study assistant to encourage me to reach the goal that my village had helped me start.

Looking back, I realize my mother had given up her shot in order to care for her family. She had given up a scholarship to Lane College, about 90 miles from Memphis, to take a job and stay home with my grandmother, who had become a widow in my mother's last year of high school. She stayed in Memphis to help support the two of them before I was born. She gave up her dream of becoming a schoolteacher and became a preschool teacher instead, which did not require a degree. After her illness and my graduation from high school, she knew it was a matter of months before she would pass, but she was determined to keep me on the path. Her strength, choices and sacrifice, until the very end, gave me the motivation and the grit to keep going, never considering other options. I had known that I would have only one shot, so I took advantage of it.

> "Like words from the play Alexander Hamilton, written years after I had lived it by Lin-Manuel Miranda, a fellow Wesleyan graduate, 'I am not throwing away my shot.' Even when things were not going well, having the God-given courage to turn that adversity into something positive is what I learned to do." – Larry

Our Impaired Courtship

"I've learned...that no one is perfect until you fall in love with them." – Andy Rooney

On our first date, we went to his roommate's jazz concert. I began my lifelong affair with jazz that night. Walking to the show, Larry rattled off every famous artist he had seen and every live performance he had attended (quite impressive to a naive girl from Kansas). My date held my hand politely and slept through the whole show! "Aren't you enjoying the music?" I inquired from my dreamy state floating with the piano rifts. I was too polite to say, "Why are you sleeping through the show, are you drunk?" As I was raving about the show, he continued to nod. I did not understand nor appreciate this odd trancelike state. In hindsight, this was the first hint of unintentional tuning out, something almost uncontrollable with people who have ADD.

I liked Larry. I thought he was quite handsome and enjoyed him when he was awake, so I accepted his idiosyncrasies as part of the package. After all, he was positive, fun, curious and a creative problem solver; in addition to being brilliant. To top it off, he was tenacious, not giving up despite his challenges with planning, time management and staying focused.

My infatuation began with Larry's spontaneity, always coming up with things to do, enhancing our whirlwind spring romance. I loved his creativity to get by with little money, living on "love." I was awed by his brilliance, explaining organic science, advanced math and physics to me, a social science major.

A Horse Is a Horse

I learned how distracted Larry could be while riding horses with him early in our courtship. The distractions never really stopped; I just chose to adjust. Before mounting the horse, I had explained that I was an inexperienced rider and would need Larry's close supervision to make it around the trail. Of course, I was given the oldest, slowest horse. That nag had a tendency to stop at every puddle of water for a drink. When he reached the stream, my ride ended. The horse did not respond to "giddyup" or the less printable terms I hurled at him. There I sat aboard an old horse in the middle of the shallow stream, panicking. My date was trailing along behind me. I thought he was being polite. In fact, he was just distracted by the scenery. When he trotted right past me, I was in a state of full, unadulterated fear. The chivalrous southern romantic said he did not see me in my predicament; he was busy catching up to his friends. A grown woman waving her hands and calling his name from atop a large brown horse did not get his attention. I earned a *self-confidence badge* that day. I had to get myself out of the stream by dismounting and leading the horse out of the water. Doing so was completely out of my comfort zone, but it was the only way the horse and I could get out of our predicament. Sure, I was completely undone that he hadn't recognized my need for rescue, yet I've never been able to stay mad at him for any length of time.

From the very beginning of our relationship, Larry and I struggled to make ends meet. We had champagne taste and a root beer budget. Oh, how I admired how Larry could make $20 last a whole week. Three movies and three days of meals cooked in a popcorn popper seemed ingenious to me, as we existed in a shared tunnel of debt. My spring romance was going over the cliff, down the well, through the fence of that new foundation we were building. February to mid-May, 1970, had been a blissful courtship with a quirky, handsome man and I was hooked.

The tall, shy man with the soft brown eyes painted a vivid portrait of himself from the 20 years before we had met. Most of his stories were sad, but colorful compared to my simple two-parent family in Kansas. His independence in managing family responsibilities from age 12 showed me street smarts and experience beyond his youthful appearance unlike the immature boys back home. Later I learned how respected for his control and confidence he was among the "brothers" in college, and I was proud because I certainly respected him as well.

I was falling hard for exactly the type my mother had warned me against, a future physician. – Audrey

Just when our romance was peaking, sharing our pasts, our weaknesses and our future plans to be together, Larry said in casual conversation, *"I am leaving for Baltimore to enroll in an accelerated medical school program at Johns Hopkins in two days."* I was speechless and on the verge of heartbreak as he finished the sentence; I couldn't believe he dropped that bombshell so matter-of-factly. Being 100 miles away was one thing, but Boston to Baltimore was just too much to imagine, let alone the way he had told me. To him, it was just something he had forgotten to mention. We didn't see each other for months as Larry made it into the program and I was still in school.

Audrey came to visit me in January of 1971. In our discussions, we always had to come to a meeting of the minds. I felt she was right for me because she would challenge me and not let me have my way. I knew I would need help along the way, and I felt she would be the best person in fulfilling my dreams. And besides that, I loved her. – Larry

My mother was not pleased to hear about the premed student who was my newest "true love." However, when my parents met Larry, she put all her warnings aside because they loved him immediately and he loved them back. Mom knew *"something"* was different about him, and he became part of our family, and ours became his first real family.

"*It only took 20 years to uncover that Larry Jones, future MD, had inattentive type ADHD.*" – Audrey

Helicopter Over Hopkins

"Audrey graduated in the summer of 1972. We got married on August 26 in Kansas City. We took turns driving my little Volkswagen, filled with her belongings and our wedding gifts, to our first little apartment in Baltimore." – Larry

Instead of the important observations of day-to-day behavior afforded by living in close proximity, we had carried on the idyllic long-distance courtship. Learning a new city together was exciting and kept us on the go instead of being still. Impulsivity to try everything just made Larry more attractive to me. Yet impulsivity and exploration didn't mix well with the rigors of medical school, especially after we got married. Being in a relationship was a distraction in one sense, as it took his singular focus away from navigating the curriculum. Larry was excited about our new life and feeling as though he had already made it, so he made some poor choices. It was the perfect storm for medical school failure for the ADD student. Between being bored by science classes, making careless mistakes and being an extreme procrastinator, he struggled to graduate from medical school on time.

Despite the challenges, Larry kept his eye on the prize even when gross anatomy haunted him, taking the course twice. Memorizing every part of the human body, retaining the information and recalling it all for various oral and written exams is a trial by fire for every medical student. Then there is the actual dissection to find each piece listed, working hours over a smelly cadaver. When his medical school promotion was delayed, that triggered a reboot of his focus. It was time to complete what he started. With me as his constant companion, encouraging him, helping him study and turning into a hovering, helicopter spouse, he graduated.

Wife and Manager

Helicopters hover. When they hover, they are usually waiting for passengers to board or disembark. Because they are so powerful, the sheer strength of the blades is loud and imposing, causing wind shear and disruption, yet hovering also means rescue in a second's notice. I learned early to hover and remained in that position throughout our marriage. Being a helicopter spouse is a bit too much like being a helicopter parent, and it became my part-time job—not good for a relationship. Instead of considering some type of counseling or educational testing, I thought I could sweet-talk Larry into doing his best. I provided the day-to-day management of our lives. I handled the here and now while he was doing his best and far more than his classmates just to keep up. Although Larry had attended an excellent college, this competition was with second-generation medical students who'd been competing their entire lives for entrance to this top medical school. For a 21-year-old spouse, "helicoptering" is generally considered toxic. For the adolescent and young adult facing academic hurdles, it can be essential. There is no time for teachable moments when the perfect storm is swirling overhead.

Each course became a study map. Memorization was a huge problem for Larry but came naturally for me. Complex problem-solving, attentiveness and executive functions are necessary to make it as a physician; each was difficult for my husband. There was little time for leisure and lots of stress. For once, we totally synced. Persistence with flashes of brilliance became our signs of progress, test by test, through basic sciences. I believed I could give him love and attention. I knew Larry needed emotional support—the kind one gets from a parent that his grandmother was incapable of giving. I thought I could take care of that too. Being a helicopter spouse would give him time to relax whenever possible. I also began accompanying Larry to study sessions and sitting up over the cadavers in the Gross Anatomy Lab.

Eating dinner over a preserved human body is tough, but any sacrifice for my man.

Conquering the work to graduate was a testament to his resilience. But, medical school graduation day was less festive than we had imagined with Ninny scowling about our move to St. Louis. She fully expected us to return to Larry's hometown, and to her, in Memphis. We were certainly happy that he was finally finished, yet we were worn out from all the effort. The fact that I was eight months pregnant simply added to the exertion of the day.

"How did we get here?" – Audrey

I'm Gonna Make it Happen!

We didn't function as a "normal" couple typically does—we weren't typical. We are still married and that won't change. However, in our "marriage agreement," we each had boundaries, territories and areas that neither of us dared cross. We operated together—for better or for worse.

Even though it was a time of rapid, exciting change for me, those years were not idyllic for two naïve kids coming from the middle of the U.S. in turmoil over race and the Vietnam War. We were both looking for companionship; I found my other half. I had high expectations for a multifaceted life full of fabulous opportunities. I planned to just figure it out and make it happen." – Larry

There were no master classes for raising ADHD children or recognizing the same behaviors in my spouse. Often, the best that I managed was to avert adverse consequences for our family. Making it happen meant a formidable mountain of "make it happens" for me. Going to graduate school, obtaining the MA and MBA, were kick-starters for full-time entrepreneurship and managing Larry's medical practice before I came home to Drew, Jay and Rob. I was constantly 'making it happen' for my guys. Thus, I was vulnerable to sliding into the enabler role too often. There's a fine line between helper and enabler, especially when I was busy making it happen.
– Audrey

Motherhood: Triple Blessings in the Midst of Distraction

"Once a person who has ADD has 'accomplished their goals,' it's time to bask in the glory, not make contingent decisions." – Audrey

Larry thought it was a good idea to enjoy the East Coast a bit more before moving to the Midwest. I was eight months pregnant with our first child, and he would be starting his pediatric internship/residency program in St. Louis, where we had no place to live.

"Let's travel along the East Coast one more time before we leave," Larry proposed. Just when the angels were lighting the way to the end of the medical school tunnel, only two terms instead of three that year, we learned that our baby was due the week that Larry's internship would begin. Maybe we should have considered packing and finding a new home in faraway St. Louis much earlier than we did. That would have required planning. But as an eight-month pregnant woman with swollen feet and a freshly burned face (learning how to fry chicken), I said, *"Sure, let's do it,"* casting my cares to the wind instead of nesting. I was counting on my 70-year-old parents coming to pack and move us, thinking it would be an easy process. Perhaps it was pregnancy brain that clouded my faculties and reasoning. I was really looking for my husband to be in charge and figured he had everything planned. After all, he had just completed Johns Hopkins School of Medicine and been accepted into Washington University, another one of the top five

medical schools. I was anticipating a smooth transition and looking forward to being a doctor's wife and mother.

From Boston to Annapolis, we enjoyed sightseeing and sharing time with old friends as we ate our way down the East Coast from lobster rolls to pastrami sandwiches in NYC. It was a romantic vacation and a good rest for both of us, but the baby clock was ticking. Two weeks before the due date, we settled down to packing and house hunting. What were we thinking? Waiting until the last minute meant there was no time to discard anything—just the way Larry prefers it. We had to take everything we owned, which was a substantial amount of furniture, clothes and goods that had accumulated over our four years of marriage. Electronic house hunting in 1976 meant using the library, newspapers, the phone book and calling long distance from our house phone in Baltimore, sight unseen. My ankles were as swollen as freshly baked hoagie rolls. I had been sitting to pack, doing my best in my bloated state. Overhearing Larry on the phone trying to find a home for us was frustrating and frightening. The process was unproductive, and Larry quickly became impatient and distracted by all the unfinished boxes and chaos.

One morning, Larry said, *"I can just drive out to St. Louis as soon as your parents arrive. I'll find us a place and start work. First babies never come on time, so it'll be a couple of weeks. Then when you start labor, I can get the first flight back because first babies take a long time to come."* He was the doctor, not me, but I wanted these boxes gone and our new home to be found immediately. However, I agreed, even though I knew better. My mother was to arrive the next day, and Larry was planning to leave right after.

Although I had agreed to him leaving my mother, me and the unborn baby in Baltimore without him, I immediately started having second thoughts. In order not to discuss things in front of my mother, I agreed to ride with him to get the Chinese food for dinner. As I squeezed, quite uncomfortably, into the car, I screamed, cried and cursed. He said, *"I wish you had told me this sooner."* And I said, *"I thought you would come to it on your own. And I'm telling you right now; you can't leave me here, nine months pregnant, with my mother."* Huffing and pouting, parked on the side of the road, he agreed he would stay. I think I willed labor that evening because Drew was born the next morning on his due date. At that time I was continuing to ignore his impaired problem-solving skills.

Drew's birth quickly solved the problem of being late starting his internship, but the rest of how to move us halfway across the country was like a whirlwind nightmare. We would face other challenges as well. Making the cut through the racial divide of segregated St. Louis City, particularly getting through the gentrification around the hospitals in the Central West End, an upper-crust neighborhood, was almost impossible. Continuing segregation based on race, a Black man, even though the man was a pediatric resident, with his Black wife, a Black son and a white dog named Wiz were not part of the plan. Larry tried but didn't find any suitable places near his new hospital. The apartment he found was located in the middle of crime-ridden south St. Louis, miles from the hospital. Once he saw the location, he got the deposit back and in hyperfocused emergency mode, he started pounding the pavement of the Central West End and located a big three-bedroom apartment down the street from St. Louis Children's Hospital, where he would work.

Once my dad arrived from visiting his family in Michigan, my parents were in charge of making the move happen. I was two weeks postpartum, had no budget for movers, my husband was in St. Louis, so my dad and our friends packed the truck and drove 700 miles.

Meanwhile, my 70-year-old mom, first-time grandmother, and I muddled through everything else with the two-week-old. We took so long trying to change the cloth diaper in the bathroom at the airport that we ended up missing our flight to St. Louis. We had to book a new flight and call Larry's Uncle Mickey to tell him we would be late, but that our dog Wiz and mom's dog Honey were on the flight and still needed to be picked up. Larry had neglected to tell Uncle Mickey about the dogs, as his response to me was, "No dogs are riding in my Thunderbird!" It was going to be 100 degrees in St. Louis, and me and Mama were spent, thinking about our little canines suffocating from heat exhaustion in someone's cargo hold. I then had to call Larry to let him know we would be in late. He seemed to take it all in stride, not understanding we were in a crisis.

At that point, I started coming back to myself, wondering, *What the heck type of universe are we living in?* Larry treated all of this as just a minor hiccup. He had now moved on to his life as Dr. Jones. He was aware in his mind that my dad and a friend were driving a truck 700 miles with our belongings. How to get it unpacked was too far in the future, because he had to balance work and worrying about our arrival, but work took precedence.

I now understand ADHD's overwhelming effects on Larry's executive functions; however, at the time, we were clueless as to why he couldn't execute our move on his own.

Adjusting to Our New Life

As a child who never knew her grandparents, I rushed to have children because I wanted them to have time with their aging grandparents, so exactly two years after moving to St. Louis we welcomed Jay. We both had plenty of distractions. Our dog Wiz was our first baby. Unfortunately, he was jealous when Drew started growing, so we sent him to live with my parents. We had to move out of our lovely apartment six months after we had made it our home. The landlord actually used our apartment as a model for selling the building as condos and decided to find a way to break our lease and sell the unit. It was a tough blow for us, emotionally, financially and physically, having to find another suitable dwelling for our growing family in the middle of winter.

In those days, internships meant long hours and short wages. I wrote off Larry's lethargy at home to his intense schedule, as he was working 60 to 80 hours a week. Always helpful with the baby, he was rarely engaged in anything else because he was understandably too tired. Inspired by the other doctors' wives who were school teachers, to make ends meet, I took a job as a substitute teacher when Drew was about eight months old. Immediately after I got into the classroom, I realized I was more of an administrator than a teacher. I kept the job because as it was flexible and a good source of income, however, I enrolled in evening classes at Webster University's graduate management program, for which I felt more suited. That lasted off and on for about two years, as I started graduate school and also became pregnant with Jay.

Unfortunately, we had taken little time to learn from past missteps, so we hadn't saved any money. Although we had beautiful furniture, we still owned our old, wrecked car, were incurring childcare expenses and were still in an apartment as opposed to owning a home. We thought we were part of the emerging "new class," but we were struggling to figure things out.

The Birth of Our Second Son, Jay

We decided on natural childbirth and had even taken refresher Lamaze training together in preparation for our next son. The day of Jay's birth, I had been in labor for at least 10 hours when the doctors began discussing the possibility of a C-section because the baby was in distress. When my husband, as our Lamaze coach and a second-year resident, said to me, *"This labor is going pretty slow; I can just run across the street to Children's Hospital, and they can call me when things change. The C-section probably* won't be *necessary.,"* I was livid. The staff attributed my screaming and cursing to labor, but it wasn't that. It was Larry's loss of focus on the imminent birth of our child. After my outburst, he calmed down and refocused his attention and realized he needed to stay with the project at hand. Eight-pound, seven-ounce Jay arrived shortly thereafter with the cord still around his neck. Now that the baby had arrived, Larry became totally focused on the new little miracle, his baby.

Now or Not Now Behavior, a Classic ADD Symptom

Reflecting back on Larry's behavior at this time I think if I could have gotten up out of that bed with the oxygen mask on my face, I would have probably slapped Larry back to attention. He should have known more than I that distress was a bad sign at that point in the delivery. Rather than participating in the complex decision making, he had wanted to remove himself right then from the problem and let the other doctors set the schedule and call him "at the moment"—in other words, when it was a "now"—of the birth. He had decided to escape and say that the birth would happen "in the future" and focus on something else, leaving the problem-solving to my doctors.

Now or Not Now behavior is what Larry had displayed during my labor. Since he was yet to be diagnosed, neither of us had a clue as to why he had behaved that way. Loss of focus on anything that is complex, combined with the person's attention gravitating to something they are comfortable with, is "Now or Not Now" behavior. This behavior is often frustrating to deal with because they see a timeline as if there were two stagnant points: *It's Not Now, so I don't have to stay here and wait. Sure, it could change at any second, but it's Not right Now.*

Later, Larry explained why he had been so stressed because of what he knew as a second-year resident about the real complexity of Jay's situation. By that time, he had been through bad births, deaths, big babies, long deliveries and other issues that we were potentially facing. He had been the doctor in rotation who had to deal with birth emergencies; being the dad who had to potentially face a personal emergency was too much for him. So going across the street was what was comfortable in that "not now" situation.

For years and years, I have tried not to be angry. Through counseling, now I understand, I've been able to go back and forgive a lot of those old wounds. If you don't, it's like a fresh burn—it stings to the touch and isn't healing. It's important to go back and deal with the pain and get past it.

The Birth of Our Youngest, Rob

The next year, our third son would be born. Waiting for Rob to arrive another crisis of childbearing arose, prepartum depression confirmed by the obstetrician. At this point, Larry was working at the neighborhood health center and doing a genetics fellowship. Now he had multiple jobs with multiple responsibilities, which meant complex problems with time management. Meanwhile, I was doing my best to take care of home. My pregnancy was hard. I was shaped funny, was more sluggish, worried a lot and literally had my arms full with two children. Jay had just started walking, and Drew was only three. I constantly thought, *"Who is going to hold the new baby?"* I only have two arms, and together, Larry and I only have two laps. Larry had to focus all his attention on his work, so functioning at home was difficult.

In my previous labors, the doctors had broken my water. With Rob, my water broke at home, and I was ill prepared for it. My doctor husband scolded me for dripping on the beautiful bedside straw rug as I was completely overwhelmed in the moment. Though Rob was early, my mom was already in place as Larry rushed me to the hospital in our low-riding rental car, as I had just wrecked our new station wagon, which was being fixed. Unfortunately, the main thoroughfare was under construction, and I felt every single bump as we made it the few miles to the hospital. Thankfully, Rob's was an easy birth, as I was in labor less than five hours.

Making It All Work Landed Me in Surgery

Rob was a happy baby, so it was easy for him to fit in. He just wanted to be held all the time. Literally, I was trying to figure out how to hold Rob constantly was a dilemma He often spit up after eating, he required feeding more often while being held at a specific body angle. As he wriggled and grew, along with the two little ones around my ankles, the weight and positioning took a toll on my ulnar nerve at the elbow. The injury caused my arm and hand to be nearly immobile., requiring surgery for correction. My parents drove from Kansas City to care for the children. During the visit, my dad repaired things around our backyard, as we had moved into our first house a few months before Rob was born. Dad decided we needed a fence and promptly ordered one from Sears to keep our boys safe.

The surgery was to be laparoscopic, a minimally invasive procedure, however, once they began the procedure, they could see the nerve was entrapped requiring a different procedure. When the doctor went to the waiting room to find Dr. Larry Jones, he was nowhere to be found because he had gone to the nursery to see one of his newborn patients. The anesthesiologist woke me up during surgery to give permission to do an invasive surgical procedure that would permanently relocate the nerve. When Dr. Jones returned, I was in the recovery room bandaged from wrist to shoulder in a soft cast that was covering staples and a very long scar. They kept me overnight because of the major surgery, but truth be told, I was a little relieved to get a little rest, if only for a few hours.

> *"At this point, any of Larry's idiosyncrasies became less important than getting through the task of taking care of three kids. Raised as an only child, I was now a full-fledged mom, responsible for taking care of a house full of inattentive, impulsive guys." – Audrey*

Becoming a Dad

"When the children are infants, that's the easiest parenting gets." – Larry, Dad and pediatrician

Drew was born June, 1976, the day I was supposed to start my pediatric residency in St. Louis. but his birth delayed my start date for two weeks. Fortunately, I let the director of the program know I was a new father, and he put me into a fairly easy rotation as we settled into a comfortable apartment in the Central West End. Becoming a father was exciting. Being an only child, having met the woman who was right for me and then bringing our son into the world was the best feeling. He slept through the first night without waking up and he didn't wake up to eat in the middle of the night, hardly ever. It was nice to have him as a first baby.

Two years and 11 days later, Jay was born, a healthy, big baby boy, weighing 8 pounds, 7 ounces, unable to fit any of the clothes my grandmother had made for him nor any of the others that were waiting for him. He ate all day and all night and whined and whimpered all through the night. I had to create some techniques that allowed us to get some sleep. One was that I would put him in a rocker baby seat next to our bed so I could get sleep. When Audrey would wake up and ask where her baby was, I would tell her, *"Right here, at the side of the bed."* He has been a night owl ever since.

I found out Audrey was pregnant with our third son in Kansas City at the movie theatre while watching *The Deer Hunter*. I was still sitting there stunned after her announcement. I totally missed the end of the movie and have never been able to watch the movie since. We were not planning to have another child that quickly. The pregnancy took me by surprise. Rob was our IUD baby.

We had moved into our first house when Jay was three months old, and Rob was born 16 months later. He was very different from the other two. He ate well but became a big spitter-upper after about 6 weeks. Evaluation by his doctor found that nothing was wrong with him. He would eat, spit up the bottle he drank, and then eat again, filling up what he had lost. We had to keep an extra set of clothes on hand for him and for us. A few months after he was born, my grandmother came to visit, telling us the baby was going to die because he was spitting up so much. That statement nearly frightened Audrey to death, so it became a difficult task to keep both Audrey and my grandmother calm. As Rob matured, the spitting subsided and the really difficult behavior management began. He turned out to be our largest child, reaching 6 feet 3 inches as an adult.

The accidents and impulsivity with our sons began almost immediately after Rob was brought home from the hospital. I remember Audrey holding Rob when Jay came in from preschool; he saw only the baby and thought his older brother had been traded in for a new model. A few days later, Drew was running to Jay to greet him as he came in, tripped on the rug and fell into our round, glass coffee table where he hit his brow. The cut required stitches, and the marks are still visible above his eyebrow even though he was only 36 months old when it happened.

> "As you can tell, Audrey's perspective is quite different than mine."
> – Larry

Fatherhood, Making It Happen

Not having a father of my own made raising my sons more of a mystery than I would have liked, but I was determined to make it happen, with flair. – Larry

I Wasn't Really Interested in Housework

My mother, grandmother, and I were renters through my childhood and adolescence. Not meeting my wife's expectations of a husband being a handyman was a problem for me. Her father was a great handyman. He would come down to help sometimes and even bought me my first set of tools. I knew about keeping up a yard, but had no experience in terms of taking care of a house. Time management was never my strong suit, and I was much more comfortable focusing on things I liked to do rather than things I had to do. Household chores got done, but little projects would take forever. They would sit for a while and then even longer, and the project would never get completely finished. Why? I'd get distracted. I would spend time doing something else. I got constant calls from patients in the evenings and would spend the rest of my time with the kids and Audrey. We went to the movies at least once a week, which was a family tradition for many years. Then there were extra outings like going to fairs or going to the park, especially after the boys were able to ride bicycles and could ride around the park. Things around the house were put on the back burner. We paid workmen to do a lot of the big stuff.

I liked the idea of being a handy dad but not the reality. Truth be told, I didn't really want to spend time on certain things, especially manual labor involving tools I wasn't familiar with using. I would rather pay someone else to fix what needed fixing, especially after we started making and saving more income. I really enjoyed the tedious things like refinishing furniture, but taking the time to do that wasn't a priority. As a kid, I didn't mind cutting the grass because I had done it with my grandmother. I knew how to do that.

We owned a lawn mower, but I paid someone to mow our grass from the time we purchased our first house. However the hedges were my domain. Trimming them was something I felt I had expertise in. I didn't want anyone to touch them. There was two-thirds acre of hedges around the perimeter of our lot. I kept the hedges in good shape, pulling out the limbs and weeds and trimming them every two weeks in the summer. We lived on a corner lot, and it was the first thing people would see when they passed our house. "When can you come and do mine?" asked a neighbor in all seriousness, thinking I was a hired worker, not Larry Jones, MD. Our house, yard and those hedges were a source of pride for me. In hindsight, I didn't make trimming the hedges a family chore involving the kids. I'd make them help me in terms of sweeping up, but that was about it, we should have cut the hedges and yard together, especially as they got older.

Maintaining Control???

That's when Mary came into our home. Thank God for Mary. I had previously worked with her at the hospital, and she agreed to keep house, tend to the boys and cook on Saturdays. She was a great advisor in terms of how to rear the children since she had come from a large family. When she came over, she brought her son Brian, who was Drew's age. It worked out well as Drew had someone to play with, and the younger two could play with each other. It also gave Audrey and I a chance to do chores and to spend time with each other during the day. Her counsel was great; she told us siblings should not fight but should protect one another from outsiders. As two only children, we needed to know this as parents. They didn't fight with one another, but stuff still got broken around the house. Throughout their lives, I adjusted my schedule to be home and help my sons get to school in the mornings. Periodically, I visited their schools to ensure they were displaying good behavior, as they never knew when I would show up. In those days, it was simple to stop by the class, peek in and check on them. We believed doing this helped with discipline.

"They never became hyperactive at school because we were active parents during their education." – Larry

Lack of Self-Control and Impulsivity Are Key Traits of ADHD

Our three sons were born in rapid succession within a three-year period. They were each gifted with (undiagnosed) ADHD, yet the way the traits affected their behaviors were different.

Drew, the oldest, was a handsome, clever, super-confident chick magnet who was like a third parent; his younger brothers revered him.

Jay was book smart and reserved in the classroom, but an attention-hungry risk-taker, always plotting.

Rob, charming, friendly, impulsive and as big as his brothers by age six, was the youngest and the first to be identified as gifted with ADHD.

Being so close in age, adventures with them were often a blur, as something was always happening in our home, even when they were young.

Locking the Door

"Grandma said, 'Don't lock the door,' but I did it anyway!" – Jay

I was three years old before I had any time without Drew's hand on me. As soon as Grandpa and Grandma Robinson drove down the highway with just little Rob and me, I knew something had changed. We had left home without Drew! Who was in charge? Me! What does in charge look like? I was a three-year-old plotting mischief. This was huge. My grandma was over 70 when I was born. This trip, I was on my own even though Grandma never left us alone. Our visit had daily tests to see how I could outrun, outhide and outthink my loving, trusting grandmother. Grandma thought all my tricks were so cute. After a week or so, I was getting bored. I needed to show her that I really was the smartest kid. Every day, Grandma showed me the lock; every day she warned me not to push the button. One fateful day, she told me that I would lock her in the basement if I pushed the button. As soon as she said it, she knew she had made a mistake! I couldn't wait! Moments later, when she had descended into the basement, she heard the lock click behind her. I pushed the button. I had to do it. I had to find out for myself if the door really locked. How could I learn if I didn't try new things? – Jay, the second son

My Son Did What?

When I spoke to my mother on the phone, she was catching her breath, somewhere between tears and laughter. My mother said, *"I'm sorry, baby, I knew I shouldn't have told him about the button,"* through her phone in Kansas City. *"Of course, your daddy was not at home. I panicked immediately, but I tried not to show it. All I asked Jay to do was to sit right there until I figured out how to get help. I couldn't see Rob from the window in the door. I was thinking as fast as I could. I could hear them banging cabinet doors in the kitchen. At least they were close by, right above my head. But I was stuck behind the locked door. I called from the basement phone, but nobody had a key except your daddy and your uncle. I finally reached your uncle at his church. You know it was Sunday, and they didn't want to interrupt service, but they could tell I was upset and sent him home to rescue us. By the time your daddy came home, it was all over."*

I felt so badly for my mother. Going out with the boys by herself was too much of a chore, since Rob ate all the time and Jay was busy. So my elderly mother had stayed home from church, thinking it would be easier to control the boys in an enclosed environment, only to be locked in the basement. I knew immediately that Jay had locked his grandmother in the basement on purpose. Then I thought of their safety. At least the baby could only crawl. I imagined daredevil Jay turning on the oven or falling off the cabinets. Before I could say anything of significance, she continued.

My mother remembered that in all the crying and fuss afterward, she must have said to Jay, 'If you don't like being at my house, go home!' It was silly, talking to a three-year-old that way. *"It all happened so fast, really baby, I'm sorry she kept saying. I left your daddy in charge while I finished the wash; he put them down for a nap so he could take his Sunday before-dinner nap too. I should have known better since Jay never sleeps at naptime. I was only in the basement 15 minutes when I had a mind to check on them. I heard the front door rattling. Jay was at the front door, turning knobs and pressing buttons. He must have been on his tiptoes to reach all the locks on the front door. He made it through the big door to the screened-in porch, but he couldn't reach the porch door's hook. As I made it to the front hall, I heard Jay screaming out to his baby brother, 'Come on Rob, we're going home!'"*

I felt so badly then to think they had tried to escape on their own! I tell you, we all had our hands full with those boys. Thank goodness my mother caught them before they made it out of the house!

After that experience, my mother made her rule: one Jones grandson at a time. I couldn't blame my aging parents one bit! Happily, each grandson visited for one month every summer for several years. Although there were no more reported incidents of outsmarting Grandma, I'm not sure what happened as she never told and neither did they. My dad taught them how to ride their bikes, about using tools and how to fix things. Together, my parents took them on interesting excursions and culturally enriching outings. Self-esteem building and identifying new interests always came from their visits. When they returned home, all of their stories were about total indulgence.

"*Being alone with their grandparents gave them something they didn't have at home—undivided attention—which went a long way.*" – Audrey

The Droopy Eye

Hyperfocusing was a way to avoid following directions, even at age four. – Larry

Jay enjoyed adult company more than being with kids. We often had get-togethers at our home. There were always built-in playmates for our children, as families attended as a unit. When the families left and our children were sent to bed, Jay would just sit up, listening to the adult chatter. He was always awake in his room standing in his crib by the window waving goodbye to the last guests.

At a holiday gathering, one of our guests was an Asian man with a droopy, lazy eye. That eye became Jay's focus for the evening. His brothers and the other children were together as a pack, and they listened to instructions as we, the adults, shooed them upstairs. Not Jay—he had to understand why this man's eye was different than anyone he had ever seen. So he followed the gentleman from the kitchen to the living room to where he sat on the couch. When Larry noticed Jay hanging around and staring, he asked, "What's wrong?" Jay kept saying, "His eye." There came a point when looking at it was not enough. Pointing his little finger, in full voice, Jay asked, "What's wrong with his eye?" The room fell quiet. No one knew what to say. His dad, never missing a beat, sternly directed Jay up the stairs, out of the conversation. Our friend laughed, as he was accustomed to people commenting about his eye. At the time, no one said anything about the rudeness of our four-year-old, and the gathering continued.

Behaving this way was not a sign of some type of budding genius.

Hyperfocus and impulsivity led to many "Oops, I didn't mean to say that" or "I just couldn't stop" moments. When he behaved this way, people would say things like, "Oh, he's so observant." No, he was rude, and it was unacceptable behavior. He didn't want to be with the other kids and would choose something, anything, to be fascinated by as a way to distract himself from whatever instructions he had been given. Hand holding was usually required to manage his behavior in groups.

> *Hyperfocus and impulsivity are a difficult combination to manage. While kids need to focus on tasks, impulsive focusing is difficult to manage. Repeated incidents of unusual behavior should be reported to the pediatrician just as any repeated physical illness."* – Larry

I Know This Doesn't Sound Funny But ...

I coped using humor; however, that was not healthy. – Audrey

I make excuses to make all the other excuses fit so that my life will make sense. If I don't, then things make me crazy. That started when the kids were very small. I had to laugh so many times to keep from going crazy. I would excuse my laughter and say, "I know this doesn't sound funny, but ..." and end up telling a completely difficult, hurtful episode in our lives to the pediatrician, at a teacher's conference or even at work, just to cope.

When I was in graduate school, I made excuses for never carrying pictures of my children. I never carried them because they were always in my head—I had the three of them. I never went to work and said, "Oooh, I made an A in science yesterday." Just having a bit of adult time away from the house freed my mind enough to go back and survive more adventures. I remember the first time I started laughing because I was uncomfortable thinking about, let alone retelling, an incident to my peers. There was nothing funny about it. Rob ran away at the annual hot air balloon race, in a park filled with 100,000 people, because he was upset that I wouldn't buy him a hot dog. Being impulsive at three years old, he disappeared into the crowd on purpose. I immediately headed to our seats on the lawn; Larry was there, but Rob wasn't. I left the other two kids with him and went to the safety tent. I gave them his name, described him and his clothes and then felt like a completely bad mom since I didn't have a picture to show. I started to break down, but I couldn't cry…I had to hold it together; I had to find my youngest son! They were looking at the Black parent who had lost the Black child in the massive crowd as if I were completely negligent and ill-equipped to mother a child. I had completely forgotten that I had given each of the boys a whistle before we left home in case they got lost. They began calling him on the loud speaker. I was so upset that it took me 15 minutes to clear my head and remember to mention the whistle around his neck. They asked him to blow his whistle. Finally, we heard his whistle. He had nearly found his way back to our seats. He was always good at finding his way.

On Monday, when I got back to school, it became the rolling joke about me not being able to keep up with the kids, but I was also sad and embarrassed. I was one of the oldest enrolled in school and had three young, busy boys. Most of my peers were right out of college, and I was about 10 years older than them. Even though I never brought the kids around campus, everyone knew about my three little boys. I always looked like I hadn't slept. I was always late for study groups or had to leave early because I had to balance dropping off, picking up and caring for them. We were just barely getting by on my fellowship funds, which included a small living stipend as Larry was just building his practice and we could barely pay for childcare.

Before becoming a wife and mother, I was a sociology/anthropology major in undergrad school. At the time, I had wanted to be a social worker. I learned through a formal internship that I was not empathetic enough to be an effective social worker. Besides, I thought being an entrepreneur would give me more time with the children. It didn't! However, I've had the life I wanted, given the cards I dealt myself because I ended up being a social worker in my home. That is the problem with me as the parent. I wanted to generate solutions to solve problems, traits which make one more suited to business. I liked the administrative issues so much better than the teen issues, which all sounded the same. Different circumstances, same sad, scary, not-funny scenarios. So when I had to recall the stories, discuss the drama or deal with the fallout, I laughed and used humor just to make it through each incident.

> "If I hadn't led with empathy, I would have cracked and fried on the sidewalk." – Audrey

Present Yet Disconnected

"Compensating with work was much more comfortable for me than dealing with the nuances of the ADD challenges I was facing internally and with my sons' behavior. Being present, enforcing rules was all I could manage to offer many days. Hyperfocus is extremely difficult." – Larry

When Rob's behavior was difficult to control, I would create more structure for him since whippings were not working. He was required to bring home a report from each teacher that his teachers and I had developed. This report had to meet the expectations set at the beginning of that week. I would say, *"We are planning on going to the fair this weekend. If your report does not meet the agreed-upon performance, nobody goes to the fair."* Fun family events were always all or none. Audrey and I agreed that we would not split the participation in weekend activities. All went or none went. The intention was to use peer pressure from the older boys to make sure that Rob did not get in trouble and to make sure that his work was completed so that we could all participate. That strategy worked well.

I was physically always at home or at work. We agreed to work hard to give our sons the best opportunities to be well educated. Family focused, we did not participate in social groups except church on Sundays. Our evenings were spent with the boys. I was busy with checking kids homework with them, bedtime rituals, and answering patient calls. Family communication was usually only over dinner, but there was little communication beyond the daily tasks.

Both of us now understand the major challenges we had faced because of my busy home and work schedule. We did not share our individual takes on our lifestyle except in the "911" moments. We never considered balance; each of us just did what we thought was our "share" of maintaining the family, we were both present but disconnected.

Faking Seizures

"Falling down the stairs became a game to him. It was as if Jay had to re-create and elevate the experience, showing early some dangerous signs of being a risk-taker." – Audrey

Jay and Rob were in constant competition for maximum attention from their older brother and us. At seven years old, Jay figured out a way to manipulate us by faking seizures.

It started out with falling down the stairs. The first time it happened, Drew was at the bottom of the carpeted stairs when Jay tumbled down from the upstairs landing. Drew was upset seeing his little brother fall because he considered himself to be his protector. Though his head was spinning, Jay quickly recovered and exclaimed matter-of-factly, "That was fun!" while his pediatrician father examined him for neurological and physical damage.

The second time Jay fell down the stairs, Drew came to his rescue since his dad and I were out and they were in a sitter's care. When we arrived home, big brother Drew reported this fall. Fortunately, everything seemed to be okay, physically, at least. By the third fall, we began to suspect that they were not accidents but intentional. Jay's explanation was that he just seemed to black out. He said he got dizzy and couldn't see anything. These falls seemed to give him some type of adrenaline rush, coupled with plenty of attention, as he began having frequent falls down the steps. It became a game for him.

Larry, as the pediatrician and dad, had a long discussion with him, explaining that falling down the stairs was quite dangerous. After that discussion, Jay would appear to pass out and only fall on the floor, not down the stairs. He would manage to fall at a time and place where Drew would discover him: in the hallway, in his room or in the kitchen doorway.

Once in the kitchen doorway was my only encounter of discovering him after a fall. The kitchen had two entrances—one by the stairway, where I was descending, and the other by the den, where the brothers had been entertaining themselves. I screamed. It frightened me to see my child sprawled out in the doorway, and I screamed again. Drew came running behind his brother, and we tried to revive him. He had, by that time, orchestrated the perfect fall, with all indications necessary to convince us that he was unconscious. As he lay there, he slowly came back to consciousness from a limp state. Drew and I picked him up and took him to the sofa as we coddled and questioned him. This was so over the top that we mutually agreed he needed to go to a pediatrician who was not his father. Our pediatrician was one of the calmest persons I have ever known and assured us that this was something that happens with children and not to worry. She told us to watch him closely and to let her know what happens. We did, and he repeated the behavior; however, he was more careful to fall unconscious only when his brother would discover him.

Drew was getting terribly upset, to the point of tears, in his concern for his little brother. These falls continued in episodes over the course of several months. At the end of the school year, the pediatrician advised us to hospitalize him to run neurological and psychological tests. We took her advice and did so.

Come to find out, hospitalization is an attention seeker's dream. Everything was focused on Jay. He didn't have to share the spotlight with his brothers; it was all about him. During rounds, doctors asked if he had a certain symptom, and by the next day, he had developed it. However, all the tests were negative. Everything about him, including his temperature, was normal. After five days, he barely had time to visit with us because he was having such a fabulous time with the hospital's amenities, including the latest electronic games. He was never in his room. We had to search the floor for him, usually tracking him down at the nurse's station or in the playroom.

On the sixth day, we were told we could take him home since he had these nonconcrete, phantom symptoms. Just before he was to be discharged, the nurses found him sprawled on the floor in a dramatic fashion, complete with liquids spilled and belongings scattered. When he came to, he explained that when he had stood up to get out of bed, he just blacked out. "Seizures" is a diagnosis of exclusion when there are no other test results indicating a particular clinical diagnosis. Therefore, they sent him home on seizure medication because of that incident. Seizure medication is dangerous for people who do not have a medical cause for taking it. The results were horrible. The prescribed treatment became a punishment to our family. He actually became sick and cried all the time, and so did I. He was nauseous, couldn't eat, became dizzy and became scared out of his wits, as did I. He didn't want to take the medicine, but, being his mother, I insisted he take it as prescribed. He wasn't ready to give up the game. Instead of admitting that he had made up the blackouts to get attention, he tried to avoid taking the pills. That strategy did not work. I felt so badly that I hurt along with him. He was even allowed to sleep with us, something the children had never been allowed to do, because I felt I had to keep an eye on him. When the weeklong regimen of medication was up, that's when the professionals told us, "Look, he's not having seizures." The doctor said, "The seizures are only in his head." The recommended course of action was to have "a strong talk with the child" about faking the symptoms. Faking an illness requiring hospitalization to be the center of attention was an early indicator of narcissistic and risk-taking behavior. With Larry being on staff at the hospital, they took the symptoms at face value. If he hadn't been a physician's child, they probably would not have done all of the workups and likely would have told a regular parent that he was faking much earlier. By getting one over on us this time, Jay aimed for bigger, riskier ventures since it was never proven officially that his seizures weren't real. In his mind, he had outsmarted us; he was "the smartest child." This experience taught him that he could invent and rationalize just about anything and get away with it. He pushed the limits to gain attention. He understood that medical emergencies got the attention he craved. After thoroughly ruling out physical causes, neither we nor his pediatrician directly addressed attention deficits. We started him in studying martial arts, hoping to work on the accident-proneness and self-discipline.

> "*Unfortunately, it's difficult to separate backfires of hedonistic behavior from scene-stealing attempts. After the negative results of seizure tests, we did not take the next step. A psychiatric workup would have pointed to ADHD and other possible problems such as anxiety, depression or a conduct disorder.*" – Larry

Creativity and Hyperfocus

"Being the big brother was a great role; however, because the three boys were born within a span of four years, Drew became the third parent and never the focus of the complete attention he deserved." – Audrey

Drew is a naturally talented artist. Unfortunately, we did not understand his hyperfocused behavior. If we had, we would have guided him differently and sought support earlier. Painting was his favorite art medium. We annually visited African American art exhibits in Atlanta as well as the local museums and galleries. Our home has always been full of artwork. After several suggestions from his art teachers, we enrolled him in an accelerated summer painting program. During the weeks of work, Drew was excited about the painting within a painting he was creating. It was to be a room with a stained-glass window. The completed project would be on a 12 x 12 canvas. He had learned to sketch and then would complete the painting on canvas. The sketch was extremely detailed. Ten classes later, at the end of the course, the sketch was even more detailed but only half of the stained-glass window was painted. We were disappointed, knowing that he must have been distracted by something. Applying his talents to developing other artistic skills led to several other false starts, like the theater internship. Drew is a natural-born actor. His first role had been in a professional production as a singing and dancing minstrel at age 12. We enrolled Drew in every type of theater program available. He knew that was his calling. He has the ability to be convincing in roles and lead with confidence and cleverness. We believed the expensive and time-consuming programs were worth the investment. While his high school grades had ebbs and flows, we were so proud of his starring roles in every theatrical production.

> *As a parent and a physician, I failed Drew by not recognizing his ADHD when the first subtle symptoms began to appear. When he was in third grade, his teacher suggested that he might have a learning disability. He could not remember when assignments were due, and he always seemed to lose homework in stacks of disorganized old and new papers. Perhaps because of my determination to see my son make it, I ignored what was said and focused on discipline and good behavior because those were things I thought I could control. Perhaps I couldn't accept that something was off because it would mean something could be off with me as well? Heck, he was my oldest son; he had to be okay, right?!? – Larry*

Video Games and Cars Are Not the Same

The ever-confident Drew couldn't wait to learn to drive. It became a major ambition by age 14. The day he crashed the front and rear of the family car at the same time with Rob in the backseat, he said he just had an uncontrollable urge to prove that he could do it—that is, drive without any instruction. As we began to observe, a pattern of overconfidence and underperformance began to emerge. The boys hadn't wanted to go into the store with me. I thought that leaving the 14- and 11-year-old in the Jeep while I went into the strip mall shoe store was no big deal. I had parked right outside, and they opted to stay in the car and listen to music. Suddenly, everyone was running outside. I had decided to try on one more pair of shoes, ignoring the gawkers until Rob burst inside crying and screaming. He had no loyalty, just hysterical tears, shouting, "I didn't do it, Mommy, I didn't do it!" As I'm grabbing my belongings and trying to comfort Rob, the other shoppers returned to the boutique, bemoaning the odd fender benders. One Jeep, driven by Drew, had managed to smash into smaller cars in front and behind it. Running outside, after assessing that Drew was unscathed, I resisted the urge to scream and slap him at the same time. Drew had a perfectly serious explanation for his antics. He told me that after a "lifetime" of observation and skillfully "driving" in arcades, he didn't need to wait for his driver's education class at age 15. He was ready to start preparing for the car he would be getting at age 16. As the third parent, he looked forward to being chauffeur to his brothers. His imagination had seized on the opportunity being left in the Jeep had presented. He knew how to start the engine but didn't realize he had his foot on the gas the entire time, as arcade games didn't jerk backward when the gear was shifted to "R" and the accelerator was pressed. Of course, after crashing into the car across the aisle, the only move was to pull back into the original space. The problem was that the same thing happened with "D" and acceleration; he crashed into the vehicle in front of him too. *"There must be a problem with the Jeep. I just put the car back in the space where I started,"* he rationalized as his screaming, terrified brother clung to me. I remember standing in that parking lot, looking at three damaged cars, without a cell phone in those days, trying to process this new complex mess as I left notes for the other drivers and piled my sons in the car along with our bumpers. Convincing the owners of the other cars to allow us to pay for their minor damages was the first step in solving the complex mess. Once settled, we faced the major damage to our own car. By not reporting it to the insurance company, we thought we were dodging a bullet of high rates for teenage drivers. This was an extremely expensive lesson of which none of us understood the consequences. In fact, we were enabling Drew to have a clear driving record when he started driving legally at 16. For Drew, this incident was just a malfunction that could have happened to anyone. Forget the facts; simply pass the problem to Mom and Dad for them to fix. Consequences were minor for him since withholding driving privileges wouldn't be a punishment since he was only 14.

What We Learned

We would have done things differently knowing what we know now. First, I would take the third-grade teacher's comments more seriously about Drew's performance at school and his inability to complete simple assignments in class that most of his classmates were able to finish. Had we taken her suggestions, we would have had him tested sooner, then we would probably have noticed similar behaviors in the other boys and started treatment before they had reached high school.

What We Should Have Done:

- Set personal consequences for paying for the accident.
- Determine the criteria for the path to a driver's license, including grades and behavior changes.
- Require completion of driver's education class and extended supervised driving.
- Develop a contract for driving privileges.
- Increase driving privileges based on merit, not convenience.
- Plan positive incentives such as purchasing a well-used car.

Teenager Alone in Paris

"Jay was a risk-taker and put himself in great jeopardy while traveling internationally with only his teachers as chaperones." – Audrey

Jay purposely refused to participate in the accelerated classes offered in elementary school by not completing the tests. He revered his big brother and cherished his friends. He did not want to surpass them in any way that may have caused resentment or separation. Of course, we didn't figure out his motivation until years later. Nonetheless, he was always an exemplary student. When he was 12, he was doing well in middle school French and was invited to participate in the annual seventh grade trip to Paris, a coveted honor many students strived to achieve. One of two African Americans on the trip, Jay traveled with a dozen students to Paris for Spring Break. The school offered parents the opportunity to chaperone. Hindsight is 20/20. Knowing our son and his lifetime of risky, impulsive, attention-seeking behavior, one of us should have chaperoned when we were offered the opportunity, but we didn't.During the trip, we received a call from the cops that he was detained for shoplifting. His explanation was that the teacher wasn't attentive enough to check with him before moving on to another store in the Paris mall. He said, "The others did the same thing." This was daring talk for a 12-year-old alone in France, as he was dramatically telling a bald-faced lie. In fact, the others were more cautious and had followed directions. As we learned later, Jay lagged behind at every stop. In the open-air flea market, when the students were supposed to be together, he stopped to make a purchase and his wallet was stolen. He ran after the man, screaming at the top of his lungs, in his best broken French, "Please just give me the wallet!!!" Eventually, the man dropped the wallet. Retrieving his recently deceased grandfather's wallet delayed the group's tight schedule. Moving from the Eiffel Tower to Notre Dame to the Moulin Rouge with Jay in tow must have been a challenge for the chaperones. But from his perspective, the teachers just weren't attentive enough to him. Jay refused to take responsibility for his actions even when he returned home. During a discussion with the school superintendent, instead of him listening or owning up to what he had done, he began tattling about the teachers' behavior, which led to the school district's canceling the program for future classes. He said the chaperones did not meet his expectations. It was a shame because they were just doing tourist activities, but the way Jay painted the picture, continuing the trips could be seen as too much of a liability, I suppose. As his parents, one of us should have been a chaperone on that trip. Thank God we were able to resolve the shoplifting incident long distance, but we didn't recognize the seriousness of this pattern of behavior as we should have. Opportunities come with risks. In hindsight, we should have never sent Jay abroad without one of us to chaperone him. As parents of children who are known to be impulsive, we must be vigilant in helping them plan by setting limits and rewarding extended success.

> "International travel involves constant, complex decisions that most 12-year-olds are not prepared to make, let alone those with ADHD." – Audrey and Larry

Impulsivity

"When impulsivity took over, Rob wanted what he wanted and placed no value or consideration on the consequences." – Larry

Maximus Prime was a main character in *The Transformers*, which had just been released. Like most popular movies, it had action figures that were all the rage. We went to three or four stores to find this 16-wheeler truck that changed into a Transformer. It was expensive and one of the most sought-after toys that Christmas season. The truck also belonged to Drew, but Rob wanted an action figure. Impulsivity took over. Before the winter was out, Rob slipped Maximus Prime out of the house to school and traded it for a $5 action figure, the Incredible Hulk. Maximus Prime had cost $40. One day, we asked where Maximus was since we hadn't seen it in a while. Caught, his face became expressionless. After we asked several times and then saw the Hulk, he admitted he had traded it. After asking whom he had traded it to, I took him to school the next day to get the phone number of the child's parents so we could exchange the items. We did get Maximus Prime back and put it away. Rob wasn't able to play with it for several weeks since he didn't appreciate it.

> *"For hedonistic and ingenious kids like Rob, it usually wasn't the same infraction twice when it came to his impulsive behavior. If your child is naturally creative, smart, strategic or a risk-taker, understand that the stakes only get higher as they age." – Larry*

What We Should Have Done:

- Tackle impulsivity with patience and steadfastness.
- Gather all the facts before you get too upset because a kid's first defense is to shut down.
- Provide the lesson to the child as to why the behavior is inappropriate and why they shouldn't do it again using real examples.
- Give consistent lessons after each incident and talk about potential situations in age-appropriate ways.
- Report recurrent troubling behaviors to the pediatrician.

Rob in Transition

"Rob's motto was: 'If it feels good, do it!' particularly when he was in the hyperfocus zone." – Audrey

Hardheaded

Always inquisitive, friendly and ready to introduce himself, Rob never met a stranger he wouldn't talk to; it was part of his impulsive personality. When Rob was three years old, he started writing on the walls in the foyer of the house—specifically, drawing pictures. We didn't know what he was doing or why. He would get into his brothers' crayons when no one was looking and start doing what he wanted to do. We tried every punishment we could think of to get him to stop, but he wouldn't. He was the most hardheaded child I have ever met, especially when he was left to his own devices. Spankings and punishments didn't work. We had a tradition of going to the *Disney on Ice* show every year to celebrate his birthday along with Grandma and Grandpa, who came to town to join the festivities. Resorting to drastic measures, we finally threatened to cancel his fourth birthday party if he didn't stop. Even that didn't work. He was so upset that we weren't going to the show that he somehow climbed on top of the kitchen cabinet, managed to fall off the edge and punctured a hole in his earlobe, which is still slightly visible today. Because he had to be the center of attention, he didn't care if it was negative or positive, so he got what he wanted that day (attention), but we held firm to our decision of no birthday party.

Boy Scouts and Bullets

The tall husky one in family pictures, Rob also stood out because of his dark eyes and bright smile. He was the best known in the neighborhood and at church. He was so big that by the time he was six years old, he and his brothers, who were eight and 10, were wearing the same size clothes! As they grew, they favored one another so much that it became difficult to tell them apart. This is around the time they started being known in the neighborhood simply as "the Jones Boys."

Being the third son, Rob was a team player who rarely complained or snitched. His brothers made all the decisions and used him as the scapegoat whenever possible, but as parents, we knew most of their games, and Rob got only his share of punishments. He also did his brothers' chores just to get a share of rewards. He was a trooper who accepted direction and exploded only periodically when physically frightened by their prepubescent, borderline dangerous behaviors.

Being a member of the Boy Scouts really helped him to transition from childhood to young adulthood. In the beginning, Rob shared the condition of most 10-year-old boys—hating to bathe. His older brothers had begun Boy Scouts together but quickly fell off. Jay flat out quit Scouts because one trip with the bugs was enough. Drew didn't like being comrades in the woods, feeling the boys were mean and played too many tricks on one another. Rob, on the other hand, flourished. He was the only Jones boy in Scouts when it was his turn, and this distinguished him. It was just the thing he was looking for. Becoming a Cub Scout and making his first trip away from home to camp was heaven for him. No baths. With little coaching, he was camping and earning merit badges, moving to each level of Scouting. Applying his single focus to Scouting and with his gregarious nature, he was group leader at each level. Rob began climbing the Eagle Scout ladder. He had a goal to complete Eagle Scouts by age 16 and by 14, he was on his way to achieving his goal. That summer he went on his last trip to summer camp, the one needed to complete his Eagle Scout application requirements. He had earned all of his badges; however, behaviors we had all overlooked almost derailed his achievement.

This was his last camping trip, and he intended to add to his "one of a kind" reputation. Unfortunately, he ended his experience with a big bang and would later try to justify his behavior, which is a classic ADHD trait. Consequences were always an afterthought. Parents and children see and remember things differently. I remember riding in the passenger seat of our little car as my husband sped up the highway to collect our young troublemaker. Larry was angry, I was upset, and we were both concerned about the consequences because we didn't know the full story of what had happened.

Rob recalls:

I had been riding the summer school bus with one of my friends. We went to his house to shoot firecrackers after school because his family had so many left over from the Fourth of July. I bought a few firecracker packs, some Roman candles and a few other items from him. I took them home for my brother Jay and I to shoot off the back deck, but that wasn't too exciting because we didn't have an audience, so I took the rest to Boy Scout camp. My buddy had some starter pistol blanks he brought to camp as well. We were 14-year-old thrill seekers and planned to set them off in the woods with other campers. We just didn't have time to get away from troop activities until the Order of the Arrow Ceremony when we were walking by and saw all the fixings for a giant, unexpected fireworks display. Kindling for a huge bonfire was set up in a clearing in pitch black darkness; after the fire was ignited, an arrow would be shot into the sky, all part of the annual ceremony. Passing casually by the bonfire site, we set out firecracker packs and sprinkled blank bullets. Night fell at camp; I'd told about 20 friends so they would be prepared to enjoy the thrill. We expected some intermittent pops during the bonfire burn, just a little extra with the crackling wood. We underestimated the thrill. One leader described 'bullets flashing past his head.' Starter pistol shells don't explode that way. But he was screaming like he was shot and on fire at the same time. It even surprised me.

The next day, the big Black kid was easily identified. Caught, as I often was, in my most elaborate productions, I begged the camp director not to call my parents, to let me get home and explain. An empathetic, kind man, he reminded me that I could lose my Eagle Scout passage. I was determined to finish my passage more than anything ever. He offered me the worst punishment, calling my parents to pick me up that day. I don't even remember packing. I just felt like I was going to death row. To this day, I don't remember the punishment. All I remember is feeling like Tina Turner caught in Dad's sports car, with Ike Turner driving. Pop, pop, pop led to pow, pow, pow!"

Upon throwing Rob's belongings in the trunk, we headed back to St. Louis. Traditionally, my husband had gone along with the kids, laughing at what they had done and refusing to be a disciplinarian. Before this incident, his dad would justify his behavior by saying, "That's just Rob." However, when the "Buddy Parent" turned on Rob, he stopped talking. With every question came an evasive, noncommittal "I don't remember" answer. As his father got angrier and angrier, he began hitting him while driving a stick shift. I was in the backseat watching them, scared for my baby as his dad grilled him. As I watched and listened, it occurred to me that something really wasn't right about Rob. I knew how important Scouting was to him, and I knew he could not have purposely, knowingly jeopardized his investment without something being seriously wrong.

Back then, Rob thought the fireworks production was fun, and today, he still remembers it as being fun. In his mind, the punishment was immediate, in the car, then it was over. It's interesting that Rob doesn't remember the months he was grounded or the real consequences of his actions over 20 years later. His actions were hedonistic (self-indulgent). Actually, they had always been hedonistic. In other words, *"If it feels good, do it."* There weren't any books written about ADHD back then in the early '90s. While my husband accepted his son as, "That's just Rob," I was not satisfied with that any longer and was determined to get him help.

> "After the incident, we initiated a conversation with his pediatrician, which began a dialogue about behaviors that were later identified as ADHD." – Audrey

Say What? ADHD? No, Not We!

"It wasn't until our youngest son was diagnosed in 1990 that our other sons and I got tested. I went through denial before embracing what had always been present." – Larry

I had never considered I may have inattentive type ADHD let alone that I had potentially passed it along to each of my three sons. I became a pediatrician in 1976. The prevailing thought in medicine at that time was that ADHD ended between ages 15 and 18. There had been a few reports of adult inattentive behaviors as ADHD, but those seemed to be for "those folks who did not fully mature." The first case of adult ADHD I learned about was one of my instructors, but the person wasn't that old, and I just let it go in one ear and out the other.

A Fellow Pediatrician Was Diagnosed with Adult Inattentive Type ADHD

Shortly thereafter, the local newspaper ran an article about another pediatrician, a colleague, who realized she had adult ADD. We often wondered about her because she was disheveled every day. She was an excellent clinician, yet it was hard to miss that those wash-and-dry suits she wore were always wrinkled. Since her husband was also a doctor and his appearance was fine, and they had several small children, we assumed she didn't have time to get around to ironing her clothes, attributing her appearance to inattention. We also recognized some disorganized thoughts, as she was at times unable to clarify what she meant. Her behavior was way off the chart, more like a child's behavior, more hyperactive. She got tested, was diagnosed, started on medication and was much more organized almost immediately. She began to understand and manage some of her idiosyncrasies. The transformation was remarkable. The diagnosis explained her appearance, behavior and communication style. Unfortunately, I didn't recognize my actions and behaviors as they related to her. At that point in time, I never made any connection with my own family or myself.

Acting Out in Class Wasn't Our Issue

In the '80s, ADHD was the prevailing disorder; its primary characteristic was inattention caused by hyperactive, impulsive behavior. The busy, hyperactive kid who can't sit still, hollers out in class, can't wait his turn or stand in line epitomized the diagnosis. That was not our children. The less obvious attention disorder characteristics of ADHD adolescents include slow reactions, quiet demeanor and inability to control their focus. Our children were well-behaved yet easily distracted. They were quick to say yes, slow to finish. This made them likeable because everybody likes kids who behave that way. When they begin to lose focus and disconnect, there's an appearance of drowsiness, an almost trancelike state. Our kids were the ones who never got detention but suffered strongly from constant excuse-making. They didn't plan or complete assignments as they were easily pulled into their own worlds. It wasn't until Drew's third-grade teacher indicated he had some short attention issues that we considered there may be something else going on. However, we still didn't get a diagnosis until several years later.

Everyone's ADHD Doesn't Look the Same

Now we know ADHD operates on a spectrum, and that was not common knowledge back then. What that means is that every case does not look the same and those affected may or may not be "hyper," which had been the "normal diagnosis" for this adolescent condition we expected people to grow out of.

It wasn't until 1990 when our youngest son, Rob, was diagnosed that I accepted ADHD was within our household. Even when he was diagnosed, I didn't consider that I may have it. However, it made me consider the behavior of my other two sons. When I took Jay, our middle son, for evaluation and his results showed he had mild ADD, I took the test right after him because his psychologist had said something about how it frequently runs in families. I had it. I was a well-established pediatrician in private practice, and I had adult ADHD. How was this possible? I was successful. Our family was something to be proud of. We were accomplished. My patients and I had excellent rapport. I was a good doctor. I wasn't dysfunctional, though I had dysfunctional behaviors. I could compensate for those at work. The attention to detail I was required to do at work never seemed to carry over to home life. I hyperfocused on the boys' studies and behavior, making sure they were socially appropriate. Other than that, things fell apart at home.

> *"The diagnosis enlightened us as to what had been happening in our home, which helped. Yet, with it, we were faced with the reality that things were not normal and we had lifelong issues to prepare to handle." – Larry*

The Many Faces of ADHD

Realizing things needed to change once we had the diagnosis, we started looking for information about ADHD. Back then, there wasn't much to choose from. Even today, experts have differing views on how to handle it. Things move so quickly, and as children age, the stakes become greater as the risks escalate. All of it is overwhelming.

As parents, and now grandparents, we live with the effects of ADD in our family and do our best to navigate the consequences. Perhaps some of these terms and explanations, simply put, will be helpful in recognizing what is happening and begin to support you in moving through the journey.

The ADD/ADHD Iceberg

An iceberg is like a mountain hidden beneath the surface. It's as if seeing the snow-capped peak is all there is, being unaware that seven-eighths of the mountain is not visible to the eye. Much like the hidden mountain, ADHD traits are often concealed, and because of that, exploration is necessary. – Audrey

Understanding ADHD Was Easier Using the Iceberg Concept

The Iceberg concept has been an illuminating tool for us on our journey, and we highly recommend it to other families. Only one-eighth of an iceberg is visible, and most of the large mass is hidden beneath the surface, which makes it dangerous if you are unaware of what's happening below. "This is just the tip of the iceberg," as a saying, means "this is the first hint or revelation of something larger or more complex." When considering ADHD, certain traits tend to be visible on the surface (at the tip), while most of them are below.

Discovering Chris Zeigler Dendy's "The ADD/ADHD Iceberg" allowed me to review Larry's and the boys' behaviors from a new perspective (Dendy, & Zeigler, 2007). The Iceberg concept made things easier to understand since Larry and the boys didn't exhibit a lot of the out-of-control, hyperactive behaviors in school or at home that had been discussed in the books by Dr. Edward Hallowell and Dr. David Jensen focusing on controlling hyperactive behaviors. Larry has always been the opposite of hyper—more a reserved introvert. His ADHD has now been diagnosed a Inattentive Type or ADD. The boys were a busy bunch who always made decent grades with few school discipline problems. How did we miss the subtleties of ADHD when struggling with Larry's issues or our sons until they were adolescents? The Iceberg showed me that there were behaviors hidden below the surface until there is a major life change, particularly for the adolescent and young adult. Some behaviors are obvious and others are not.

Obvious Behaviors

These ADD/ADHD behaviors are often repetitive. Our boys' behavior was situational as their stories show.

Common Hyperactivity and Impulsivity Behaviors We Saw:

- On-going lack of self-control
- Quickly denying obvious behavior
- Poor recollection
- Quickly defensive and losing temper
- Constant arguing with siblings

Inattention Behaviors in Our Family:

- School problems, including:
    - Poor reading comprehension
    - Poor memory of technical facts
    - Poor homework comprehension and completion
- Poor organization of everything
- Distractibility
- Interruptions in family discussions

Not-So-Obvious Destabilizing Behaviors

These symptoms were challenging to identify. The most obvious results that we have seen in our family were: disorganization, incomplete tasks, poor decision-making and excuses.

Weak executive functioning included:

- Fear of complex problem solving
- Unable to separate advice from criticism
- Difficult to unpack complex problems to develop solutions.
- Rationalize rather than accept responsibility.
- Defensive, emotional responses

Impaired sense of time meant:

- Only two times: right now and sometime in the future (Now or Not Now behavior)
- Chronic lateness due to loss of time
- Difficulty discussing and planning long-term projects
- Impatience with others timeliness

Sleep disturbance

- Waking up late for school
- Waking up late for work
- Late night rambling
- Falling asleep uncontrollably

Difficult-to-Understand Behaviors

Initially, we just believed that these were personality differences between us. The punishment usually did not matter, especially to Rob. Larry now admits that he rationalized his behavior just like his sons..

Not learning easily from rewards and punishment

- Ignoring rules is irresistible
- Managing behavior is based on personal reward and punishment system
- Making decisions without considering past mistakes
- Expecting immediate rewards for any behavior changes.

Difficulty controlling emotions

- Short fuse/loses temper easily
- May give up more easily/doesn't stick with things
- Speaks or acts before thinking
- Concerned with own feelings
- Difficulty seeing others' perspective

According to Zeigler and Dendy (2007), these behaviors are often closest to the root of the ADHD issues and are the most guarded. ADHD is more complex than we realized. We had only focused on school problems. We did not associate Larry's behaviors with the boys' diagnosis for years.

Relating these behaviors to what is happening in your family helps; however, keep in mind that it's just a start. In our home, our sons' impulsivities had not been malicious, and they displayed a reasonable level of civility, kindness and love that were expected in our home.

The Iceberg gave us the framework we needed to put things together. We had weak executive functioning and developmental delay in our family, which meant difficulty resolving complex problems and making poor choices, to say the least. – Audrey

What We Learned

- Relating what's happening in your family to documented behaviors helps to change the focus. However, keep in mind that it's just a start.
- Impulsivities may not be malicious if the child also shows a reasonable level of civility, kindness and love toward others.
- The entire behavior spectrum may not apply to your child.
- Therapists may suggest testing for coexisting mental conditions or other serious learning disabilities.
- Figure out what to do with the information, skills and resources you have available.
- Acting on signs and symptoms as early as possible may reduce college and career derailments.

Nothing Is Normal

"When they were little, minor incidents mounted. As our sons grew, there was always something going on to keep us off balance. We were always teetering because of the effect of unexpected behaviors within our family." – Audrey

Before knowing we had ADD, we never had a holiday without incident. Something always tipped the apple cart. Every time we thought we had effectively dodged a bullet, something bigger happened. And as the boys got older, the stakes got higher. We also responded quite differently. Larry felt overwhelmed, saying, *"ADHD is like riding on a constant roller coaster in the way behaviors affect those in the household. For us, having four people affected kept the whole house teetering. As things continued to be chaotic, Audrey, the only non-ADD person in our house, continued to inflate the bubble, saying, 'Larry, you should have done this, you should have done that.' When she criticized the moves I made to provide discipline, structure and normalcy in our home, her words fueled my frustration."*

I felt that their father, the man raising sons, should be the disciplinarian and should provide the structure. As a girl, my mother did it for me, and I expected Larry to do the same for his boys. As things continued to be chaotic, I realized my husband really had no training. My own father was the only example Larry had. We both struggled with our emotions, dealing with the boys and their antics, working together daily and maintaining our sanity and marriage. Many days, it was a struggle, but there was no time to deal with the pain or frustration because something else was always on the horizon.

It's important to share the intricacies of ADHD with the diagnosed child, not just sharing a term or labeling them. One thing we learned not to do was to "lean on the diagnosis," allowing it to define the Jones men. Once there is a diagnosis, it's best to approach those gifted with ADHD with understanding and work through what's happening, seeing what you can do together. Labeling doesn't help; planning and working together does. The diagnosis helped us muddle through. Learning that each male in our home was affected by ADHD at least answered the question of what was amiss. Knowing gave us a sense of relief and allowed us to reflect on the past, and to sift through the current messes we faced daily. This was an opportunity to connect behaviors and a diagnosis, and to begin to do something about it.

In the Midst of Chaos

It's easy to think, *Is it me? I must not be a good parent! What did I miss?* As they get older, getting more frustrated with the antics is normal. It's easy to get in a panic, but it's the behavior you want to interrupt. To keep thinking it's you, what you did or did not do, is counterproductive. Beating yourself up, living in a constant state of guilt or trying to control everything does not work. You must choose to focus on what the person is good at—not what they aren't. You must support them and their natural talents, working with what they have been given and encouraging that. Focusing on "you" as the parent is ego driven, and you must shift away from that. Men, especially, need to remember that.

> "Until the day Jay told me, 'It's not you, it's me. Until I want to do it, I won't do it,' I lived in a bubble of worry, shame and wonder, feeling so many times that I should have done something different. In reality, I didn't know what I should be doing." – Larry

Building a Village for Our Sons

"Recognizing that we want the best for our children but cannot do everything for them, we welcomed support and guidance from others who cared about us all." – Audrey

Raising awareness about ADHD and how it affects schoolwork, higher education opportunities and, ultimately, workplace performance is critical for maturation at every stage. Once we figured out what was happening, with the learning problems and maturity, we were able to get relief by focusing on plans to increase success and productivity. For us plans included counseling, structure, active participation in church activities and essentially building a village to support the boys in their academic and extracurricular endeavors.

Parenting three African American males, we taught them to be courteous, obey the law, respect everyone and always do their best. We ate plenty of meals together, attended church regularly, and supported each son's interests and activities with love and empathy. Thank goodness for all the people who supported our family. We adopted an "it takes a village" mindset, finding the right people to make up for the areas in which they needed support. Our reality was that we were both hardworking parents with lots of moving parts. We were each growing our own businesses and supporting each other's. By the time Rob and his older brothers reached high school, it was a diverse crew of parents, church members, friends and staff populating our village. As Drew and Rob skated (with bumps and bruises) through their less challenging high school experiences, we thought we were climbing the mountain of generational ascension. When immature behavior and poor executive functioning rose above the surface, we honed our skills as enablers. Sometimes it was easier to fix the problem than participate in problem-solving with our three sons. We didn't have the luxury of time for in-depth evaluation of the long-term versus short-term behavioral consequences; we just fixed the issue and moved on.

Though the Youngest, We Learned About Rob's ADHD First

When Rob experienced an early meltdown in ninth grade at a parochial prep school, we were directed to an excellent, innovative educational counselor who was also a certified behavioral assessment examiner. After multiple discussions with her and his teachers, the "Below the Iceberg" behaviors began to show patterns. The academic challenges were not so much related to typical inattentiveness as to his constant momentum, in which he never stopped to absorb the work. He hyper focused on Eagle Scout project steps but forgot about the multiple long-term class assignments. Rob had difficulty determining how much time was needed for everything from completing homework to answering test questions. There were two times: *Now* and *Not Now*. If he didn't understand the assignment, he was too frustrated to ask for help. Things he understood like art, foreign language and music were great. Math, English and science, particularly lab classes, were often too challenging to attend. He was disgusted to lose his place in the school choir because of his GPA. The counselor conducted a variety of tests and interviews with teachers and with us for the behavioral evaluation. Ritalin was becoming popular as the "one-size-fits-all" solution for learning and behavior issues, but we didn't go that route. With an equally whopping financial investment required, it was not the average path for African American children, but evaluation was necessary as far as we were concerned. As we were completing questionnaires for Rob's evaluation, we started to think about behaviors that we had excused as "boys will be boys" over the years and recognized that their repeated behaviors and them not learning from rewards and punishments had been clues pointing us to these diagnoses.

We described Rob's norm as:

- Impulsivity
- Intrusive behavior
- Lack of hindsight
- Needing immediate rewards
- Stubborn
- Forgetful

The evaluation process was particularly helpful and insightful. As the mother and wife, I recognized this immediately as my life, realizing I had been living with the ADHD traits in my husband and in each of my sons. Because these were not his father's norms, as a functioning professional, Larry did not relate the behaviors to himself—it would take a while to get there. One of the greatest benefits of the counselor to Rob and our family was pulling our village together. She taught Rob to focus, successfully complete tasks and comply with the rules. Mastering this was key for his ultimate good. For example, Rob was allowed to take an untimed ACT test instead of a timed one because of his diagnosis. His score increased from 22 to 28. When he started working with the counselor, he was able to channel his creativity to solve problems outside of school too. These life skills were crucial to his ultimate career goals. Had she not asked him questions and encouraged him—without this village approach linking our entire family to developing projects based around his interests—he likely would have continued to flounder.

In addition to the school successes, our greatest rewards were learning the positive mirror traits of negative behaviors that Rob learned to apply.

- Impulsivity = creativity, curiosity
- Intrusive = gregarious, eager
- Stubborn = persistent, hyperfocused

We found the book *Superparenting for ADD: An Innovative Approach to Raising Your Distracted Child* by Edward Hallowell, MD, and Peter Jensen, MD, tremendously helpful in understanding how to support and guide our sons as the process of dealing with ADHD unfolded.

It was a tough school year, but Rob learned to combine creativity with:
- Time management to complete projects;
- Behavior control to avoid time-wasting punishments;
- Focusing on long-term goals versus immediate gratification; and
- Learning to analyze mistakes to improve outcomes.

We were helicopter parenting our children so much that we treated them "the same" once we recognized that each of them had Inattentive Type ADHD. Let's face it—we didn't know any better and did the best we could. The problem with that is simple: Each child is different and has different needs, issues, interests and areas where they excel and where they have shortfalls. Of course, all these years later, we can see what we did wrong. For that, we owe the boys an apology. If we were to do it all over again, we would not have done everything for them. They didn't learn some of the crucial life skills, survival skills or critical thinking skills that would have prepared them for a higher level of maturity and perhaps better decision- making. Had I understood earlier, I think I would have started to explore help. Since I didn't have a clue about their or my own ADD, it was easy to encourage hyperfocusing on schoolwork and activities because that's good. Interest in the opposite gender is normal as teenagers age; however, hyperfocusing on girls, that's not good. Having an understanding and working with each child as an individual would have helped them to develop coping mechanisms and behaviors to counteract the effects of the ADD. For example, with our oldest, I would have helped him nurture his interest in drama club as he was an excellent actor. In general, we hadn't noticed how good each of them was in the arts. Therefore, we didn't use those activities as incentives or bridges to remain engaged and disciplined while being creative.

> *"We didn't understand how coaching them to pursue those interests could help with productivity, self-esteem and successful moments in addition to accountability, responsibility and maturity." – Larry*

Build a Village of Educators and Others Who Support the Adolescent's Goals

Thankfully, today, learning and behavior disorders attributable to ADHD are delineated from every point of view in books, articles and on the Internet. A competent counselor will require parents and children to complete multiple inventories and a battery of tests to develop an individualized treatment plan for each child. If a counselor suggests a "one-size-fits-all" plan, starting with medication, **move on!** As ADHD is often familial, like ours, as a parent, the introspection may be uncomfortable to complete, but it is necessary.

Zeigler Dendy offers four steps:

1. Work in partnership with school officials and teachers.
2. Address academic issues first.
3. Educate school personnel about ADD or ADHD.
4. Change the environment…if needed.

Kisha Holden, a member of the Morehouse Medical School faculty, has defined the effect of the village in the African American culture in landmark minority health disparities research: *"Spiritual and religious practice as well as the role of the extended family are important sources of emotional, social, and material support for ethnic minorities"* (Holden, K., et al., 2014). However, academic and social developmental delays in African American and Hispanic children are unfortunately overlooked more than twice as often. Dr. Gail Mattox of Morehouse (2014) observes that parents have poor information about ADHD, including the potential racial stigma, potential for drug addiction, lack of access to educational and medical resources, and costs of special services. Denial of issues is a major factor that is only addressed when legal concerns arise. Some denial, she notes, blames ADHD on "too much sugar intake." If you believe ADHD is affecting your family, don't allow your personal bias to hinder getting the needed support.

Our Church Family Provided Foundation for Our Village

One of the best things we found in St. Louis was a church home. We joined our church in August 1978 and have been a churchgoing family unit ever since. As parents, we have felt blessed by angels throughout these years. Our Christian upbringing and faith, one of our common bonds, has always been the springboard for our successes and the safety net beneath our lapses in judgment and being lost in parenting. Our theme song begins, *"Through it all, I learned to trust in Jesus."* Having such a small family here in St. Louis, we relied on our church family to support us and we supported them as well. We were all able to serve at many different levels. Our children made lifelong friendships; as part of every youth group at church, the boys flourished through the love and relationships they shared. The people with whom we attended church and school functions, we treated as though related by blood. Being involved in holiday programs, camps and retreats and becoming youth leaders were a big part of their lives, just as it had been for us when we were growing up. We also sent them to parochial schools because we felt that education should be faith-based. As parents, this was one of the best decisions we have made because, even as adults, they have an anchor in their experience as Christians.

> *"People can be smart and educated, but there has to be glue, knitting them together. What's the glue? It's got to be more than lifestyle. The glue is shared and mutual faith."* – Audrey

He Didn't Remove the Pins

"Fifty percent of all teenagers with attention deficits have trouble falling asleep and waking up." – Chris Zeigler Dendy, M.S.

We thought that all high school–aged boys existed on vampire time. Each had a separate clock, which did not synchronize with the family's hectic morning schedule. We just knew that they had no routine and stayed up late on school nights doing homework at the last minute and/or working on the project they had "forgotten" to list in their school organizers. *It was the '80s and early '90s, and organizers were the way we kept track of information before computers and cell phones.* Another tactic for avoiding bedtime were the late-night searches for the assignments they were sure they had completed earlier. Jay's homework was always the first to be checked, but he was usually the last to fall asleep. Anything and everything could stimulate him for a few more minutes. To his credit, he was often reading or assembling something without using directions. He would even stay up to wash and iron the white dress shirts he was required to wear to school. On weekends, however, there was a standing contest to be the last out of bed in the morning.

Now we understand that sleep deprivation is particularly harmful to students who already have specific learning problems like solving complex problems in advanced mathematics or in life. No one was taking ADHD medications, so that was not the cause, as many seem to believe about the medications today. All of our family members with attention deficits had difficulty sleeping and waking appropriately. Their dad led the pack in staying up late, having difficulty waking up and rising on time. Mornings were a four-man marathon. Instead of two coaches, there was just one—me, the mom and wife—as I was also preparing for my own workday. Unfortunately, lots of snapping, screaming and harsh words were the start of most school days.

Being the smartest and most prepared, Jay panicked one morning when there was no clean white shirt for school. He actually liked the prep school uniform of white shirts and ties. But in his morning "walking dead" state, there was no clean shirt. Sometimes plans went awry—that was life—but he didn't respond well to the dilemma. Drew would have solved the problem in one of his normal creative ways, such as washing the collar and cuffs to wear it a second day. Not Jay. His solution was hasty instead of creative; it was risky and resulted in jeopardizing his health.

Dr. Dad describes the event:

Keeping the wound a secret was easy for Jay. He just went on about his day. His arms probably started to itch and swell during the day. By evening, both arms were red and started to look like Popeye's forearms. The long red scratches just below the arm crease were a warning; however, he didn't show us. For Jay, it was no big deal since he had been able to put on his new white shirt without pressing it. It was his lucky day as far as he was concerned.

By the next morning, he was slightly feverish but still hiding the cause. He self-diagnosed flulike symptoms. We left him home and reported his absence. By noon, a painter working in the house tracked us down at our jobs. Jay was in pain with a high fever and seemed delirious. I left my patients to go check on him as Dr. Dad. I'd seen the remnants of many children's accidents, but never this before. In addition to the fever, his arms were hot to the touch. Both arms were cherry red and tender to the touch. Each was continuing to swell like expanding balloons on the front sides of the elbows. The situation was serious, so I took him to the ER. As we arrived, I felt that I should have been a better parent to protect my sons, and I was also embarrassed going to the same hospital where I trained and sent my own patients.

Those thoughts lasted for just a few moments as I refocused on what was important—saving my son's life.

The ER doctor examined Jay and asked for an explanation of his injuries. To our bewilderment, we heard the short version of how he had put on his shirt for school the previous morning. He had found a brand-new shirt in the drawer. He was frantic trying to get dressed. So he unfolded it without removing all the pins and managed to scrape himself with those pins on both his arms. Since there was no bleeding, he proceeded on to school. After the examination and hearing the story, the physician called in a consultant who asked a few more questions. Jay repeated the same story. Quickly, the wound treatment moved to a new level. The ER staff was very concerned because of the severity of the swelling, redness and his 102-degree temperature. Nurses, direct hospital admission, blood cultures and IV antibiotics all in place, my colleague briefed me that it might be a blood-borne infection. They were able to rule that out after a test. However, they discovered it was staphylococcus (skin infection), a rapidly growing and virulent bacteria—the lesser of two evils. His arms were being eaten by the infection caused by the pins as his muscles and tissue deteriorated to liquid and puss before our eyes. With Jay under anesthesia, his surgeon performed an incision and drainage procedure to remove the fluid from the pockets in both arms. Because the surgeon had to drain so much fluid from the wounds, each empty space had to be filled with several yards of gauze to prevent reaccumulation of bloody fluids in the holes. The smart kid who wrote off the injury as collateral damage in a new quick-change process awoke to heavily bandaged, immobilized arms. He was lying there with blurry eyes like saucers. Jay was at the beginning of a painful rehabilitation.

Unlike his previous hospitalization, he could barely feed himself or use the restroom alone, but after four days, Jay was discharged. He was still in pain but also seemed relieved to have missed some boring classes. Not such a bad deal except that he had to make up the work and be confined to home for at least another week, with daily nursing checks. After that, he thought he would be back in action with a dramatic story to tell of his bravery.

I'm so sorry, baby," was my response to Jay after I learned what had caused the problem. As his mother, I felt horrible and responsible for not having a clean shirt ready for him. When I examined the "predator pins" that had harmed Jay, I went into guilt mode. After all, I had purchased inexpensive, "Made in China" uniform shirts by the dozen for Jay and Drew. Perhaps I should have laundered, ironed and hung all the new ones instead of giving them to my 15- and 17-year-olds to manage.

Once home, I nearly fainted the first day when I saw the nurse open the incisions,. She pulled at least two feet of gauze from each of Jay's arms. It was horrific, the gauze looked and smelled like bloody, half-mummified body wrap. I just couldn't imagine the holes in his arms or the pain he was suffering. Daily, the nurse removed and measured the gauze because she had to make sure she removed every inch that had been previously inserted. Jay and I both cried the first couple of days.

> *'I was in a hurry, and it seemed like a good idea,' was the stance Jay took about the incident. Yet he never correlated the injuries to impulsive behavior. What happened was risky, and he probably felt really smart, at the time, experiencing a type of adrenaline rush. He almost lost his arms, but he blames it on the pins."- Audrey*

Samurai Swordsmen

"Covering each other's tracks was more important than the lies and risk of more punishment, resulting in 'team' narcissism." – Larry

Being only 16 months apart in age, Jay and Rob were always vying for attention from us. ADD traits contributed to the sometimes physical and verbal battles royal. Both were self-centered about being favored over the other. Anything requiring family cooperation usually ended with hard feelings. Among the two, we had few compromises. As parents we spent too much time refereeing. The two revered their older brother, who passed all chores to them. But by seven or eight, Rob was larger, though younger, and that made it worse. Rob, being a hedonist, seldom gave in to Jay. He didn't care about his brother's feelings or possessions. Rob would destroy his brother's new toys before Christmas break ended. As they grew into adolescence, the only agreement was to cover each other's tracks and keep us in the dark about their individual adventures.

Larry's Account

We were home on a Saturday evening. We had finished dinner. Rob and Jay were supposed to clear the table and fill the dishwasher. The usual bickering about whose turn it was to do dishes followed. As parents of teenagers, we were on our way to bed by way of Saturday Night Live. I suddenly heard a loud yelp from Rob, and I knew something was seriously wrong. I ran downstairs and found Jay holding Rob's right hand. Rob was on the floor lying on his stomach. As the former Boy Scout, Jay was correctly applying direct pressure. I took one look and saw the gash on the back of Rob's hand. No one was excited except me. Jay continued to apply pressure. Since I had been the instructor for the required first aid training for the troop, I knew he was capable, but both of them were overly calm. Stoic Rob didn't complain of any pain.

I was already back upstairs dressing, telling Audrey to do the same. We were doing the emergency room drill that we had begun to perfect. Next stop, ER triage desk. Being a physician on staff at the children's hospital usually reduced the child abuse/negligence questions. No fractures, but Rob's totally limp right hand did peak the ER doc's curiosity. What happened? "I fell down on my face holding the knife and cut the back of my hand. You know how clumsy I am." Rob stuck to his story each time he was asked. Jay was right at his brother's side and even held his brother's hand while he received numbing injections before the sutures. All of the tendons on the top of his right wrist had been severed by a sharp knife we had recently purchased. In total parent mode, I was alarmed that my child couldn't raise his fingers above his wrist! I actually rationalized that it could have happened as he had explained. In doctor mode, I knew better. When falling forward, we naturally brace our hands, so I knew he was not telling the truth.

The ride home was tense as I was able to find pediatrician mode again. Both of them stuck to the same story. Less tranquil now, disturbed by the bandages and the pain, Rob just wanted to forget the whole event. For both of them reflection on the night's events was painfully real. As much as they tried to blur hindsight, I continually questioned them. The rest of the weekend was bizarre for us as parents since Jay and Rob stayed in perfect harmony.

To see Jay taking care of Rob's chores, helping him dress and cut his food was surreal even in our traumatized state. Where were our boys? Rob didn't seem to be in any real pain. But we knew that our youngest might be facing a permanent disability. I remember waiting for Monday to schedule an appointment with the plastic surgeon.

"What happened to your hand, son?" asked the surgeon. Rob stuck to his story even though Jay was not at his side. "I fell down on my face holding the knife and cut the back of my hand. I am kind of clumsy." The doctor said his hand was cut in the flexed position. His tendons were stretched when severed. The tendons snapped back up his forearm. This would have been impossible if his palm had been pressed down. Rob maintained his story. The doctor also said that the chances for reconnection of the tendons and the return of the full use of his hand seemed possible with the right plastic surgeon and extensive physical therapy. The expert was leaving for mission work in a few days.

After many prayers and before the surgeon's international trip, we were in the pediatric preoperative room awaiting the master surgeon. By now my pediatric training and experience had covered the parent hysteria. I knew what didn't happen and so did the surgeon. Rob, much too large for the pediatric furnishings, sat in the parent's rocking chair. What we thought was just anxiousness about his first hospitalization was a flood of regrets for his behavior. "I think I better tell you what really happened." He explained why he was covering for Jay. Jay turned 16 that summer. He was enrolled in a competitive STEM course that would lead to a scholarship at the state university, but being the "smart one," he had decided to reject the opportunity by not completing the course since it offered no immediate rewards and boring classes. Since Jay was already in trouble because of the summer program, he didn't want me to get any angrier with either of them. After his "Scouting beat down," he feared for the immediate punishment for this latest incident. Jay was skating on thin ice with us, locked down for the remainder of the summer, so that's why the almost 16-year-old was emptying the dishwasher at 10 p.m. on a warm summer evening.

Rob had never considered the long-term effects of his injury, just getting past any short-term punishment. Rob explained that they had been playing with knives like they were samurai swords, one making gestures toward the other and bouncing back and forth as though they were fighting. Accidentally, Jay sliced his brother's right wrist. The accident scene I found was staged as an afterthought to cover up the truth. Rob had a high pain tolerance. He had played ball with a fractured finger and hiked at camp with a fractured ankle. So Jay thought he could clean up the scene before Rob "screamed" and alerted us. The entire complex tale was concocted to avoid perceived punishment.

Even facing surgery, Rob didn't see the incident as a big deal, but for the first time, he was frightened. Reflecting on the entire debacle, he never admitted that it was a bad idea. Finally, we had a true description of the accident. We felt it was an equal-fault accident. With the full information and the expertise of the surgeon's hands, the reattachment was successful. When we returned home with Rob's bandaged, throbbing arm, we thought the surgery and the recuperation would be punishment enough.

A long recuperation and rehabilitation was ahead. This event changed Rob's life. We call it the silver lining blessing. Yet we were so busy worrying about the fighting that we didn't focus on the cover-up that could have resulted in Rob losing the use of his hand. Looking back, it's amazing the lengths they went through not to tell the truth. In the short term, their cooperation and being on their best behaviors were amazing. At last, we thought, they were changing. The cooperation continued as Jay worked with Rob on his recuperation. Probably out of guilt, he devised ways to support his brother. Of course, Rob took advantage by playing helpless. By the beginning of his freshman year, about six weeks after the incident, Rob was just beginning to use his right hand again. Unfortunately, once school started, Rob's freshman ego kicked in and Jay's hindsight about seriously injuring his brother gave way. The sibling support yielded to the old sibling rivalry; low empathy, inability to compromise and difficulty getting along permeated our home once again.

Rob had to do physical therapy, along with occupational therapy, to learn again how to button his clothes, feed himself and write. As his mother, I became his concierge and chauffeur, and boy, he would lay it on.

The reattached tendons did not a recovery make. His fine motor skills would have to be retrained. Being able to move his hand after the removal of the final sutures and bandages was reward enough for Rob. He figured the rest would come back in time. Doing daily hand exercises prescribed by the physical therapist required too much attention for the easily distracted Rob. Three days a week, we drove to the special hand therapy unit. During the ride, the conversation was usually the same. "Show us your exercise record," I'd ask him, knowing that we hadn't seen him working on them except to do normal daily activities. The plethora of excuses used to cover poor time management, not sticking with a task and his need for short-term rewards flowed as we drove from school to the hand therapist. "I just didn't have time; I'm tired after school; it doesn't help; I can write with my left hand just as well," Rob repeated.

Thankful for hand movement, we were pleased that he was somewhat ambidextrous and could type most of his schoolwork. But seeing the once-nimble right hand dragging along saddened us. He had just started to channel his impulsivity into serious artistic projects.

The Silver Lining

Molding impulsivity to creativity became the silver lining of the samurai sword experience and the path to complete recovery of his right hand. Rob learned to manipulate his hand by practicing making jewelry. He fashioned knots that became the patterns for his first earrings. Even though it meant sometimes painful repetition, it became fun just to envision and then produce a new design. First done in string and then in silver, the exercises made sense to his brain because he related them to his design work. At first, designing earrings was something to do with his time and to practice the exercises. However, he didn't share his talent outside the family. In the early '90s this was not the project to share at his macho prep school.

For Rob to complete tasks, he required immediate rewards. In the beginning, using his hand and getting positive feedback in therapy were enough rewards to begin a repetitive process that didn't seem rigid or out of his control. Molding his impulsivity came naturally to him as he was designing the jewelry. Each pair of earrings was different because he refused to copy the same piece and Rob was not afraid of mistakes because it was his work. He started his own jewelry business, which gave him income throughout his five years of college without needing to take a summer job. He continued the jewelry business as a part-time career for 10 years, winning awards and developing a national customer base for his business. He should have called it "Silver Lining."

What We Learned: Recognize excuses and cover-ups

It is challenging to recognize and acknowledge ADD behaviors as something more than boys being boys. We started to understand that grades reflected attention to school work, not a lack of understanding of the subject matter. Distractive, impetuous group actions were used as cover for report card problems.

The main lessons learned from the samurai swords incident:
- Do not take your children's explanations at face value.
- Use your best interrogation skills, one child at a time.
- Relate to your children with your own past experiences.
- Do not accept their juvenile rationalizations.

In this case, we took their explanation at face value. As a pediatrician, Larry did not use his patient interview skills. With complete information about the injury, we could have saved several expensive office visits and scheduled the repair immediately.

Repetition is an early warning sign

As parents, we often overlook those "cute behaviors" when our children are little. Those same behaviors become "ugly" as they grow and become physically adult-sized. Low tolerance of one another is unacceptable among siblings as they mature and each finds his own path. As parents, it's our job to support each child equally and closely work with each to address behavioral concerns as they occur. This includes coaching them through successes, failures and interactions with one another. Critically, what we should have done was address the sibling rivalry.

What We Should Have Done:

- Temper tantrums and emotional reactions occur but must be addressed in acceptable ways. Denying and minimizing to cover for siblings becomes dangerous as they mature.

- Rewards and punishments must be distributed equitably. Establish punishment expectations: "If you do this ..., you get this ..." in an age-appropriate manner. Communication is key in family conflict resolution.
- Adolescents must be held accountable for repeated self-centered, selfish and defensive acts.
- Family conflict resolution requires age-appropriate communication skills and methods.
- Childhood rivalries can extend to adult estrangement; therefore, addressing them early is crucial to the overall family well-being.
- Appreciate the child's natural gifts, talents and abilities, defining success based on effort. In other words, value the individual and measure his success by his level of effort and interest.

"ADD, particularly as children mature, is a force to be reckoned with. As the boys matured, we met mature versions of traits one behavior, one incident at a time. We did not fully understand their impact on our sons' maturation." – Larry

The Jones Wrecking Crew

"Four ADHD drivers at one time on our insurance policy was scary and expensive." – Audrey

We lived through this experience firsthand, first with Larry, the distracted medical student before he was diagnosed, then with each of the boys. Along with the gift of ADHD, as drivers, they typically have high rates of accidents, speeding tickets and other traffic citations.

For Drew, Jay and Rob, driving under the influence of ADHD traits was the norm. There had always been minor accidents with their dad's unusual driving style, particularly driving on vacations. Even though he swore that his heavy eyelids did not cause the swerving in traffic, keeping him awake was everyone's job. Larry had taught himself to drive, in his first car with a little help from his med school roommates. His family never owned a car, so he did not learn to drive as a teen. The first accident was one week after he got the new car on his way to medical school.

The year before Drew was born, his busy medical student dad was rear-ended. Unfortunately, the car's fiberglass body had cracked in half when he was rear-ended, causing a chain reaction upon impact. A drunken guy on the corner, seeing an opportunity, had fallen from his perch into the street, rolling under our damaged car. Larry had gone into bedside mode, leaving his car and the offending driver for the police to manage. The offending driver should have received a citation; however, Larry skipped the complex mess to do the familiar—patient care. By the time I reached the scene our car had been towed by the city and the perpetrator had skipped. Of course, the injured drunk and the witnesses were also gone. After Larry's procrastination of completing insurance forms, once he finally had turned them in, we learned the state law. Multicar pileups without citations issued became "no fault." This meant that our low-budget insurance company refused to replace the vehicle, which was never safe again. Drew spent the first three years of his life riding in a stylish car with strange cracks down both sides.

Family trips often turned into orienteering adventures. Before GPS, reading maps became everyone else's job, but it was good to have a Boy Scout onboard. For the boys, it was always more fun riding with dad than with mom. Their dad often drove erratically while changing music. He preferred stick-shift cars, and he would constantly adjust mirrors and his seat position as he shifted instead of adjusting them before driving. Because of the many distractions, he would make last-minute lane changes to exit the highways on road trips. Larry made a habit of stopping by a famous Kansas City rib restaurant on our way home from visiting my parents, crossing the state and eating a slab of ribs while driving to avoid boredom. Of course, he was always late for everything, so speeding was necessary and appropriate in his mind. His speeding tickets in high-performance cars always kept our insurance premiums above average. Observing their father's driving did not set a stellar example for our sons. He didn't change his driving habits until the burden of the Jones Wrecking Crew on our insurance premiums caused him to be obsessed with counting ticket and accident points.

A Brand New First Car

For Larry cars were a status symbol of his new lifestyle. He was a self-taught driver and car buyer. Since he missed the parental training about purchasing cars and auto care, a vehicle's looks took precedence over its value. He seldom sought or accepted advice on how to drive, maintain or own multiple vehicles, so he passed onto the Wrecking Crew his cobbled-together practices: Get in and drive the most expensive car you can afford, and always start with a new car to avoid maintenance. Thankfully, these practices have changed with age and medication.

When choosing a first car for teens, reliable, safe and used are the criteria for most. Not for this family. Because we always liked the new and innovative, we had owned the Mazda 7 that literally broke in half, the Saab that spontaneously combusted three days out of warranty and a new kind of car from a new company, the Saturn SL.

Drew successfully became a licensed driver at 16 under his dad's tutelage—he never did take driver's education. Junior year he was appointed chauffeur for Jay and Rob so that he and Jay could drive to school and manage their after-school schedules. When we made this decision, it was to relieve us from all that comes with shuttling kids back and forth, especially since Drew and Jay went to the same school, but Rob was enrolled in another. Larry had two offices and I had two jobs. Today, we understand the perfect conditions we were setting up for multiple accidents, speeding tickets and all types of erratic driving. However, we had no idea then.

No different than the expensive double crash when he was 14, Drew didn't have a sense of responsibility for his actions in the car, even though he took ownership of the car immediately. Like father, like son. He had been trained by an inattentive, impulsive, speeding driver. Second, we had established an expectation for Drew of parents funding his escapades. All tickets were paid and accidents covered. His job was student and chauffeur, so he didn't have time or need for an actual paying job since he had no responsibility for paying for his tickets and accidents. Third, my husband and sons set a precedent for their youngest brother, who years later was arrested and sentenced for moving violations in the city. When he reported to the jail, he was sent home for time served. Thankfully, the police let him go, as they said they needed the space for "real criminals." However, letting him go resulted in him not learning lessons and more serious car issues down the road.

After many confrontations about moving violations and parking tickets, Drew just hid them. He avoided punishment until the tickets arrived as warrants after not being reported to us. His weak functioning in taking responsibility for his actions was compounded by our quick fixes.

I was definitely uncomfortable with his driving, but led by Larry, we continued to be in denial, acting as if the repeated, costly mistakes were normal. Drew and Jay didn't work together effectively to schedule riding together and using the car. We began to referee their disagreements rather than focus on the longer-term changes in their interactions. Girls didn't help. Drew remained a distracted driver. These behaviors followed him until he was purchasing his own vehicles into his 30s.

Drew's first major accident was, of course, blamed on Jay since he was riding shotgun. This denial is actually more memorable than the multiple-vehicle pileup they were involved in. After school, driving in their favorite neighborhood near home, always preoccupied Drew, was hit from the rear and then hit the car in front of him. Although he was inattentive, in this instance, since he was hit from behind, he couldn't have avoided the accident. However, it just piled on to everything else about his driving and his habits. We didn't want him driving our cars, yet my husband didn't want his sons to ride the bus. As parents, we yelled at the kids, but there was little change and we didn't take their car away. So the little Saturn was repaired.

Second Son, the Risk-Taker, Gets Licensed

Frankly, we were excited to see Drew off to college so he would not be driving, since he would not be taking a car to Washington, D.C. Jay was 16 and ready to take the wheel. Being "the smartest," he whizzed through driver's education, ready for his turn as chauffeur to Rob and family errand person. Unfortunately, he decided that the role extended to all of his friends too. Gasoline was included with the car, so he was the free chauffeur for all of his old friends and newfound ones too. Drew was more protective of the Saturn itself; Jay used it as a friend magnet.

While Jay was not the typical inattentive type ADHD driver, he was a risk-taker. An attentive driver, he was always volunteering to help with any driving task, but in combining the chauffeur and risk-taker roles, the Saturn had parking violations far beyond our standard routes. Following in Drew's footsteps, he avoided the fuss by ignoring them until the license tags could not be renewed because of parking tickets. Then his big wreck happened. "After all, it was just another fender bender," Jay said. "Drew had lots more than I had," he tried to justify. He was simply picking up friends for a rehearsal. Although he had eaten dinner at home, they all wanted some McDonald's. Long story short, they didn't end up at rehearsal, and the Saturn was literally attached, bumper to bumper, to a parked Cadillac on the lot. Jay continued blaming everyone else, not taking responsibility for his own behavior. That was the end of the Wrecking Crew years. Finally, the doctor said, "No more Saturn for the Jones Boys." Pristine from the repair shop, I returned the Saturn to the dealer, where they gladly bought it back. With the Saturn gone, using our cars became a guarded privilege for Jay. Having lived through his dad's and brothers' driving adventures, Rob didn't bother to get a driver's license until his senior year of high school; he preferred to be chauffeured.

Young Adults and Alcohol—A Dangerous Combination

The dangerous, frightening scenarios of destroyed cars and/or injured offspring are occasional nightmares for any parents whose children miss curfew. Having experienced the reality twice, involving all three sons, is haunting.

By the time Drew left for college, we all knew that he was an easily distractible, inattentive, speeding driver who did not learn from his past accidents. We just did not have a name for the collection of those traits at the time. After returning home on summer break, having dealt with college trials, he was seeking new thrills. Drinking added to the potential for new levels of fun. Add into this scenario the buddy dad who had missed all that in his youth and became a willing enabler. Their weak executive problem-solving traits collided. Dad and son decided that Drew should take his dad's prized black Dodge Stealth to go to a concert downtown. The Stealth, with its sleek design and high-performance engine, reminded me of the Batmobile. The fact that his father allowed him to use it still boggles my mind. To avoid my veto, he and his buddy quickly left home before I had returned. After partying and drinking, by God's grace alone, Drew came home uninjured and no other cars involved. Unfortunately, Drew had left the car dangling from a viaduct, a mile from home, totaled. I asked Larry why he had let him take the car. The answer was classic: "I didn't want him to wreck the family car because we were going on vacation the next day."

Drinking and the Park

The summer Jay returned home from his freshman year of college, Drew also returned home to attend college locally and Rob had started driving. A fresh used car was available for Drew's job and shared transportation among the three of them. Drew was soon off to marriage. Jay and Rob were back as rivals and partners in crime. Their last auto caper gave us a strong memory of the dangers of impaired driving.

> *"The fire that destroyed our car in the park? Mom and Dad got a call from the Mounted Police who were helping us after Jay hit a tree in the city park. Because we lived in the gated neighborhood adjacent to the park, they called our home rather than detain us. Okay, we had had a few drinks. Then we rear-ended a car at the edge of the park. But being clever and more frightened about having one more accident, Jay took off into the park. I must have fallen asleep; it's too painful to remember. I just recall waking up on the way to the police station, seeing the car smoldering against a tree." – Rob*

We remember:

Three in the morning, we received the dreaded call; our sons were at the police station nearest our home.

This happened to be the Mounted Police Station in the city park. First, the officer verified their names and addresses. Second, he explained that there had been an accident, but our sons just needed transportation home, so we drove to the park to get them. The smells of vomit and alcohol overpowered the odor of horses in the large barn that doubled as a station. They could have been charged with underage drinking, driving while intoxicated (DWI), leaving the scene of an accident and reckless endangerment of the other driver. Instead of the expected drama caused by two young African American males in custody, they were just patiently sitting, waiting for their rescue. No release was required as they were not detained.

But the right address, in our upscale neighborhood, likely influenced the decision to release them to us, their parents. Thinking about this, I realize how fortunate they were that the situation did not escalate to physical harm or worse.

We followed the horrible, vile sight and smell of vomit as Jay led us to the car, still smoldering against a tree. The car was totaled, with the door panel on the passenger side dented and difficult to open. He explained:

> *"On the highway near the park, we collided with another car, driven by a young white girl. I told her we should get off the highway and pull into the park to exchange information. That was my first thought, but then I got a better idea. Since our house was across the park, I just figured we could lose her in the park and escape to our house. Rob didn't even know what was happening because he was still passed out in the passenger's seat. One quick turn, and we crashed into the tree. The car ignited. Rob was still out for the count and didn't move. I had to rescue Rob from the burning car–see, he's okay!"*

That little used car was gone, there was no possibility of an insurance claim, and it was a horrible experience for everyone. Rob was a nerd. Jay let him drink and party with the big boys. They basically received a pass for their actions; walking away unscathed allowed for more excuses and enabling down the line. Every parent can fill in the blanks of the short-term actions and reactions. We try not to recall them. For now, no more shared cars. The Jones Boys were back to lowly public transportation.

Impaired Driving

Their varying levels of knowledge and inexperience impair all adolescent drivers. Driving requires complex coordination. Texting, Snapchatting and tweeting only add to the equation. Adolescents using GPS directions to navigate unfamiliar roads miss signs and hazards and make erratic moves.

Our accounts are only a sample of the exploits of the four ADHD drivers in our home. Reflecting on our experiences, we understand layers of poor decisions that anyone can identify. However, these decisions are commonly repeated today in the more complex driving environment.

> *"Core ADHD deficits pose serious implications for driving safety." – J. Marlene Snyder, author of AD/HD & Driving: A Guide for Parents of Teens with AD/HD*

What We Should Have Done:

- Recognize and address symptoms and signs of ADHD traits early with children.
- Follow the recommendations of professionals. If medication is suggested, make a decision about its use before considering driving. I'm sure we could have saved thousands of dollars if we had related their ADHD traits in school to other major teenage activities like driving.
- Every young driver should complete driver's education. One reward is the reduction in insurance premiums.
- Uninsured driving is a guaranteed disaster.
- Denial of repetitive behavior does not change or correct the situation. Connect the dots. Adjust schedules, responsibilities, etc., to reduce opportunities for mistakes.
- Parents should share their own adolescent driving trials, both mistakes and lessons learned.
- Examine any accident calmly, determining causes and repair options.
- Set boundaries for recreational driving. It is a reward and privilege to use a parent's asset. The expenses of outings should be shared by parents and adolescents.
- Unreported and reported traffic violations should result in driving privilege suspension until they are paid.
- Public transportation is always an option.

The Last Family Vacation

"Without considering their hormones, impulsivity or propensity for creativity, we gave our sons their own hotel room one level away. Equipped with spending money, plenty of charm and freedom to come and go as they pleased, we gave them the perfect opportunity to blow it." – Larry

We were distracted, busy and unsure how to navigate all that came with raising our sons, especially as they matured through adolescence. On the one hand, we saw them as talented, intelligent and creative. On the other hand, by the time of the diagnosis, we knew some of the problems we were all facing but didn't quite know how to deal with it. We continued to make mistakes. We did everything wrong for our second offshore family event, a weeklong excursion to Waikiki, Hawaii. The trip was too long, too uncontrolled and provided too much freedom for our sons who were 16, 17 and 19 at the time.

My mother once decided to leave my father, so in 1958 she took me from Kansas to Pasadena.. The separation lasted three weeks. Since we had visited Disneyland just 3 years after it opened in 1955 and every other park in southern California with my godmother, I thought vacations were part of the Black Cinderella's life. So our sons, the little princes, had what they deserved, more than their striver parents. – Audrey

Rob remembers:

As usual, I was caught up in the plans and the punishment whether

I was part of the manic good times or not. As teenage boys, we were not seeking out danger per se, but we were more than willing to push the limits in order to have a good time. Jay and I were closer in age, so we looked for girls together when we were at home. Drew and I were farther apart, so it was unlikely that we would be meeting the same girls. However, whenever we were in a new place together, Jay and I knew that our older brother was guaranteed to get us invitations to whatever. Although we made plenty of other risky decisions without him, we followed our big brother to the ladies. Attractive young ladies were on the menu, and we had plenty of opportunities to talk to them, especially since we had Drew, the chick magnet, leading the pack.

Jay and I followed Drew's lead this time in a new place full of gorgeous teenage girls. There were plenty of girls who, like us, had come with their parents to the national medical conference, but they were boring and not exotic. There is a certain pattern to other doctors' kids. We knew there were plenty of those same type of girls from home, but we were looking for more. In Waikiki Beach, we quickly started exploring places where bikini-clad local girls hung out. We broke away from the pack in search of local color, flavor and memorable experiences. I was a bit limited in time because I was determined to keep my work and focus on my preparation goals. The new me, being compliant to my promise to my counselor to study for the ACT college aptitude test, spent time in our hotel room, only coming out with the family for the boring parties at night. Jay had finished his summer precollege camp, and Drew was on his way back to college, so they were unrestricted and in full-time meeting and greeting mode.

First, Jay and Drew used Drew's driver's license and all their spending money to rent motor scooters daily. Pretty quickly, they met two attractive local girls. I don't think they knew their ages but assumed we all were about the same age. Their adventures included scooter rides up Diamond Head, acting like the characters in a Gidget movie. Hearing their day stories nightly, I was living vicariously through them. We all stayed out late because Mom and Dad hadn't given us a curfew. One night after dinner with our boring group of doctors' kids, Drew had arranged to party in our room while our parents were on an evening cruise. The local girls showed up at our room at an appointed time. Drew had procured the liquor, and the girls seemed to be glad to be with all three of us. Sixteen-year-old me was disappointed that there were only two hotties, but they knew how to make a party. As my big brother knew, I would soon be knocked out from the alcohol.

So, I missed the sex…asleep on a cot in the corner.

Professionals leave after the 'party,' but I think these were local girls just out for a good time. I woke up after sunrise, and they were still tucked in with my brothers. I knew my parents are early risers and immediately got nervous about the scene. Each brother and his date were in their beds in some state of undress. Time was ticking, but being the outside man on the cot, I didn't say a word. Then there was the knock at the door. My problem-solving skills said to hide them anywhere. My brothers said, 'Just a moment'—a bad decision. Dad unlocked the door with his key. Again, time for them to hide, but suddenly we were all in that same space, and it was tight. In fact, they just let it happen. We seldom offered a strong defense when caught up over our heads. Drew spoke up with his typical denial defense, saying that nothing had happened. Caught red-handed, that didn't work this time. I had a pretty good fantasy about their evening, but I was mum. Not co-signing Drew's story, I invoked the 'don't tell' pact. All three of us were in a precarious situation with two unregistered women in our room. It didn't really matter who made the impulsive decisions—we were all part of it. We barely knew their names. We could have been accused of rape or anything else. They could have robbed us or our parents, whose room key was labeled and next to ours on the table. That was some bad decision-making that, as usual, Mom and Dad cleaned up.

Twenty years later, I know I should have warned my parents about my brothers' new friends before that night, but I did not. The only real punishment I remember was canceling family activities for the rest of the trip, that is, no nice meals or family excursions. It was our last family vacation."

What We Learned:

Our sons pushed the limits, and as parents, we did not limit or even monitor what they were doing, caught up in our own activities and feeling that their proximity was sufficient. We should have established curfews and check-in/report-in times, and we should have monitored their spending and activities, at the very least. Reinforcing mature, safe group decision-making and also establishing consequences of poor decisions.

- We did not have serious curfews and check-in/report-in times.
- Battles can be physically, mentally and financially costly. Sometimes the consequences or potential harmful consequences that the behavior creates topple any positive parenting model.
- Anticipating behaviors depends on past experiences and resolutions of problems created. One size does not fit all; every individual has his/her own style and challenges.

What We Should Have Done:

- Defiant adolescents constantly push limits, therefore penalties must be meaningful and memorable
- Consistently established curfews and check-in/report-in times.
- The financial costs of harmful behavior must be shared with adolescents, as part of their own short and long term financial planning.
- Always anticipated behaviors, worked through problem solving together, intervened and followed up with tangible consequences when boundaries are crossed.

With Age and Time Come Bigger, More Complex Problems

"We struggled to overcome the behaviors of our grown sons and our own addictions to helping, enabling and problem-solving. The risks were greater and the stakes were higher. Something was going to break; we just didn't know it would be Audrey." – Larry

Sex

"The use and effects of sex is different for each person gifted with ADHD." – Audrey

Father at 16?

Jay was sensitive and recognized he and his father's similarities. He loved science and math, but when it came to completing the courses, they both lost interest. He never could have a girlfriend because, in his opinion, no one was nice enough. That all changed when he met Leah. Jay always had one best friend at a time. But this time, he violated that and picked up a new, second friend, John. Leah was John's cousin, and together, they made Jay the mark by setting him up. Inexperienced in sex at the time, Leah seduced Jay at her house. Although he never confirmed the full story, we know from his description at that time, the seduction was unprotected, unplanned and unexpected. Of course, he was flattered that this pretty, experienced young lady would take time for him. Leah told him she was pregnant a couple of months later. As parents, we were oblivious as he procrastinated in telling us.

Returning from a college-scouting trip, Jay turned to his dad and said, "I don't know if I'll be interested in going to this school; after all, I'm going to be a father." This revelation happened in the dark of night 100 miles from home. Larry didn't stop driving. Instead, he conducted a two-hour interrogation in the car. When they got home, Larry told me about the conversation. What ensued was an in-depth inquisition of our 16-year-old by me. Jay had nothing to offer. All he had was fond memories of the one-night stand. He never even got a second interlude. Without her address, since her cousin John had conveniently led him there before he vacated the premises for their privacy, we were all clueless about how to properly proceed. Being the *Enabler*, I called our attorney first thing in the morning and asked, "How soon can paternity be determined?" She said, "Is the baby born?" I told her "no" but wanted to know if it was possible during pregnancy. Back then, you had to wait. The attorney said that the girl had probably received family services support during pregnancy, and if so, we had the right to ask for and get a free paternity test once the baby was born. Dreadfully, all we could do was wait.

No one heard from Leah for months. There were no baby shower invitations, family introductions or shared prenatal classes. One day, I answered the phone and the person asked for Jay without saying who she was. I told her he was outside with his dad doing something and couldn't stop, asking to take a message. To that she replied, "This is the mother of his child." I said, "Just a moment," and called him to the phone. I told him to get all the pertinent information including her full name, phone number, address and the baby's date of birth. By that time, even Jay realized he had probably been duped since he hadn't heard from her for such a long time, but we had to be sure. With information in hand, we got the paternity test and found out for sure that Leah and someone else were the proud parents of her bouncing baby boy. For somebody who seldom had hindsight or reviewed situations, I don't think Jay stopped using condoms for a very long time. However, condoms didn't stop him from getting caught up in a college tryst.

Countdown and Launch to College

Entering college is the turning point from teenager to young adult. ADHD in the 1990s was considered a childhood condition that maturity improved. The following stories about our sons show that is not true. Today, we know that ADHD teens have a longer maturity cycle. This was confirmed by Drew's and Jay's crashes when we launched them into diverse, large universities. They were functioning as teenagers but not ready to live independently. The helicopter parenting that worked in high school was impossible over hundreds of miles.

"Because we were living with the myth that financial support equaled preparing our sons for college, we were just waiting for their motivation to kick in. After all, we had made it, so we thought that the 'apples shouldn't fall far from the tree.' My distraction and hyperfocus blocked me from remembering the village that supported me even after losing my mother. Unfortunately, Audrey abdicated to me the critical preparation for Drew and then Jay for moving out of state to go to school. Since they were launching so close together, perfect storms were created, devastating both of their academic experiences at the same time." – Larry

College in Washington, D.C.

When Drew was 15 we were at a memorial service when he pulled out his wallet and a condom flew out; it went flying halfway across the room. At that point, I was both embarrassed and proud. Although secretly happy that he was using protection, I was dismayed that he was sexually active at 15. That experience made us pretty confident that when he went away to college, he would continue to be responsible. Ever popular with the girls, he had an adoring high school entourage and was a role model to his younger brothers. We all saw Drew as a leader. When he chose to attend the prestigious, historically Black college in Washington, D.C., we never once doubted him. In fact, we were proud and happy he would spend his undergraduate years in *Chocolate City*. The problem? When the big fish from the little pond got engulfed in the bigger pond, he had a meltdown. He didn't go to class, missed appointments with everyone, including advisors and teachers, and even got locked out of his dorm because he didn't pay his dorm fees, even though the money was in his account. He had become totally focused on his social life. Unlike back home, Drew found himself without adoring fans. Without others to lead, he became self-focused, oblivious to what others thought. Out of his element, he reverted to an area he was quite adept at maneuvering—ladies and sex. With this as his focus, he found a young lady to turn his attention to.

They say, "boys will be boys," and of course, teenagers naturally have raging hormones. When you have athletic abilities, good looks, charm, along with ADHD, and are living on campus unsupervised, sexual urges and tendencies can easily take over. Being "in love" can be intensified, especially when hyperfocus is one of your prevailing traits, which was the case for Drew. And when academic defeat and insecurity prevail, sex is often used as a substitute. The idea of conquering women drives the ego and replaces, temporarily, the lost self-esteem.

Being a Ladies' Man

Drew was enrolled in school for three semesters, not consecutively, before returning to St. Louis permanently. It was clear to us that he had lost a bit of himself while he was gone. Instead of going deeper or working through his challenges, Drew used his newly acquired skills in the charm department to successfully and quickly meet, attract and bed the women who caught his eye. Even with his unique ADHD gift, he attracted women and drew them in, knowing how to use his intuition to tune into their needs. He became excited about the littlest thing he had in common with a girl to show how "in sync" he was with each one, finding the commonalities to close the deal. Being creative, impulsive and completely self-absorbed, he was able to get what he wanted, quickly. While the start was clearly superficial, the consequences were long term. Sometimes he was the manipulator, and sometimes it was the new lady. Either way, his intuition was incorrect. Sadly, unprotected sex became the byproduct of his quick connections.

Long-term enabling leads to having children who are adults functioning as if they are children. We continued to be convinced that our firstborn was talented with great personal charm. But we saw the long-term effects of that profound meltdown. Back home, he did not successfully complete a semester of community college. His mantra became "college is not for everyone." He wasn't willing to put in the work, time or focus to do anything complicated like studying or attending class, and he refused to take responsibility for his actions. Even when we found a counselor who had experience with ADHD, Drew avoided the sessions with him. Living back home, taking advantage of our connections, he cruised through internships and jobs after returning to the haven of our house and enabling behavior. In his mind, he was just preparing, like the moth, to soar on independent wings. He was just in need of another chance to become motivated. He told us repeatedly, "I just need a safety net, to get myself moving." What we provided was the bridge between childhood and adulthood, enabling him to function only as an adult child.

College in Iowa

Jay decided to attend school in Iowa, a top school for engineering. We didn't realize it had made the Top 10 list of party schools. Having earned a full academic scholarship, he was one of 10 African Americans in undergraduate. With only 15 more in the school of engineering, young men like Jay were a rarity on campus. Each visit home that semester, he painted a picture for us far from reality. Assessing our expectations, he talked all about perseverance in those tough courses. But when we didn't receive his first semester grades, we learned that he had blocked permission. Something was amiss. By the time we pieced together what was happening academically, Jay was off on an impulsive romantic escapade. It was a shocking exposure of beneath-the-iceberg behaviors that tanked his scholarship. Finding a friend with benefits was a major score for the 18-year-old. At least the pregnancy scare had cut out the no-contraception behavior. However, she was a manipulative, immature girl functioning like an independent adult because her parents could afford it. Still a high schooler living in St. Louis, she pulled Jay from his studies in Iowa.

She was lonely, and Jay was willing. First, he made an unexpected visit home for Valentine's Day, at her expense. Though we were surprised he came home for a social visit, and knew it was beyond his finances, we didn't know how deeply they were falling. Evidently, they continued their long-distance love affair, and the culmination of the catastrophe was the Easter Sunday when he showed up at home in a taxi looking like a frightened puppy. Jay had managed to spend two weeks away from college, shacking up in a St. Louis hotel with the high school senior without us knowing. With sad puppy eyes and a few tears, he explained his worst impulsive decision. His new girlfriend was so lonely that she had convinced him to spend time in St. Louis at a hotel with her. He thought he was smart enough to skip a few lectures. Though he brought all of his books on the trip and had access to computers, it never occurred to him that attendance was determined by answering questions in lectures and lab groups. He cleverly had his dorm room phone forwarded to the hotel room and thought this scheme was an example of excellent project planning and implementation. He was only hurt when her parents found out the details and sent him home in the taxi without even a word to us, his parents.

Obviously, this had been his worst plan yet. Instead of reviewing the consequences of not attending classes, which had been spelled out repeatedly in orientation and first-day sessions, Jay escaped the overwhelming freshman workload in a top engineering school. He hit the wall that most adolescents meet in college the second semester. But with complex problem solving skills he did not address academic problems with a college professional or us. Instead he rationalized his academic missteps as aiding his depressed friend. After all, it was near the end of the term, so he just started the study period early, ignoring his standing in his critical pre-engineering classes.

The next day, after he arrived home in a total state of bewilderment and we went into enabler mode, the three of us went to Iowa. The experienced counselor, who he had also neglected to see regularly, asked for an explanation, Jay said, "I thought I would start final's study week early." The counselor asked one question, "What about the required attendance at martial arts classes?" Martial arts would have probably been his best grade. He had no answer and seemed oblivious to the consequences in that moment. All of us were frustrated and emotional. Too much blaming, shaming and more bandages. We left that meeting knowing he could take his finals, but that he would be on academic probation at the end of the term.

We didn't make it a teachable summer. With the lack of self-control and impulsive behavior displayed, we should have negotiated or imposed conditions for his return to college. We did not. Consequently, Jay did not return to school the following semester.

"We were relieved that summer the girl was out of his life without any other consequences. He was allowed to complete the semester. Instead, of focusing on supporting Drew and Jay to define their own problem solving plans and life paths, we continued to make one size fits all decisions. – Audrey

What We Learned From Rob's College Experience:

- Larry, Rob, and I benefited from his brothers' misfires and crashes in college.
- We understood his gifts and challenges from earlier diagnosis, and embraced the advice of his educational counselors.
- Living at home and attending a small university, Rob had advocates and family to monitor his progress and get him back on track when spurts of ADHD behaviors derailed him.
- When necessary, he used ADA accommodations.
- Rob was able to express himself and won awards as a jewelry designer while managing college. He won a loyal following as a DJ. After four and a half years, he graduated and began a career in technology sales.

What We Should Have Done:

- Research together college choices that have programs that support their career aspirations and goals, based on their strengths and weaknesses.
- Share honestly parental experiences about challenges to surviving campus life.
- Coach teen to design the ideal college for himself.
- Negotiate with the teen to choose potential colleges whose requirements they meet both academically and socially (e.g., community college, university, trade school).
- Guide the teen's final decision based on the family, financial considerations and other limitations.
- Evaluate opportunities for ADA accommodations.
- Prepare both physically and mentally for the separation if

leaving the home community.
- Negotiate communication and performance monitoring plans.
- Establish a contract with rewards for milestones.

Pregnancy

> *"ADHD teens begin having sex a year earlier than their peers. Their relationships are shorter in duration, and they are less likely to use contraceptives."* – Dr. Russell Barkley, Taking Charge of ADHD: The Complete, Authoritative Guide for Parents

On Drew's 23rd birthday, while I was cutting his birthday cake in front of the family, Drew announced, with his most dramatic flair, the results of impulsive sexual behavior: an unplanned pregnancy. I remember freezing, standing there with a large knife about to serve the cake. When I snapped back, I carefully cut and served each piece as he discussed their future together. My husband and I immediately launched into enablers. We did not ask about their plans. We knew he didn't have any money or a full-time job. We had met the mother of his child a couple weeks before. She was a part-time student. In doctor mode, Larry was talking about the due date and the pregnancy while Drew was moving the discussion to the cost of their own place, all in front of the family who knew most of the story. It was awkward. We never really talked about our feelings with him after the initial shock of the announcement.

He created the situation and fully expected us to be the safety net—to assist him and her financially. That month he said he was "getting his life together in a theater internship." How should we have responded to Drew's clear expectation for help? It was our first grandchild. His salary didn't support him, so he lived at home. Of course, in hindsight, we should have handled things differently. And yes, it was our first grandchild, which clouded our judgment! We again moved to enabler suggestion mode, encouraging them to think about parenting vs. marrying. Their relationship had been very quick, and we didn't want them to add a quickie marriage to the already complex issue of parenthood.

Then we gave them options. Stay with us until the birth, stay with us longer term until they could afford to live independently, or move into their own place with our support. Of course, they chose the last option, moving in together and marrying soon after their son's birth. We even threw in a wedding reception with all our friends to furnish their apartment and a baby shower.

The following year, there was another grandchild. She knew that the loving grandparents would ante up. Life was already overwhelming for Drew with one baby and a wife to care for. After the second baby was born, they went through quite a bit of drama, and Drew ended up with a failed marriage. He moved back home with us and soon his children came to live with us too. The young lady had grown tired of single parenting with a small child support check and was fine with leaving her babies and Drew in our care. The responsibilities of a long-term relationship and parenthood are often too much for the ADHD brain to handle. We did not like our relationship with Drew as Enablers, because of the expectation of our support for adult-child behavior, but we blamed ourselves for being too busy to see the beginning of a consistent "game." Crisis intervention is seductive. How could we stop enabling in the middle of rolling chaos? After all, enabling is an addiction.

When our grandchildren were three and four, living with us along with Drew, we found out about our third grandchild. That relationship was so short that we never met that granddaughter. We love our grandchildren, and we cherish their privacy, so to protect them, let's just say that Drew bounced, with them, between our house and his "next new love." When that relationship didn't work out, he was without a place to live, unbeknownst to us. One night Jay called in a reserved panic, saying, "I just wanted to let you know that Drew had a serious foot laceration and we are in the ER." More casually, he explained that Drew had been staying with him and his girlfriend for several days. "Drew told us about some problems he was having at his apartment with his girlfriend, so we took him in, but he can't stay with us," Jay stated emphatically. By this time, Jay already had been divorced and was in a new relationship. He didn't want to mess up his new love by enabling Drew.

When our grandchildren were nine and ten, living back with us again, we learned of grandchild number four. The children were told to keep the secret from grandpa and grandma about their new sibling. Impulsivity, lack of maturity and not learning from the past created more lives affected by Drew's behaviors. Life has given us our wonderful grandchildren. Even though Drew is now living independently with his children, it's unclear to us what he has actually learned from the failed relationships or turned away from self-focus. We are certain that our enabling only fueled his choices. We absolutely love, cherish all of our grandchildren, and do our best to provide healthy support for them.

The Enable Table

"You don't learn from the mistakes of others or your own. Those with ADHD tend to repeat the same things." – Audrey

We put pressure on our grown children by attempting to manage their families. Our unrealistic expectations were based on the way we thought our adult sons should act, look and operate. We figured they should strive and achieve to live like we did. Though ADD was a factor, we never saw it as something that couldn't be overcome. With more effort, with more time, with more passion, they should be able to accomplish their goals, be self-sufficient and amass wealth. They were "just a little behind on the maturity curve," is what we told ourselves and them, as we continued to be Enablers.

Enabling happens across the board, so the *Enable Table* game is not necessarily associated with ADHD or any other behavior disorders. However, for us, ADHD was part of our reasoning for continuing to enable our sons. We knew they were impulsive, inattentive and had trouble making complex decisions, so we just helped them. They were easily frustrated when they had to make complex decisions, so we continued to make decisions for them.

What Is the Enable Table?

Seductive and addictive for all players, the *Enable Tables* is a mind game played between the parent and the child. The more parents help and protect, the more they become addicted to the action, just like some first responders. The more the children are spoiled, the more they become entitled. Crisis intervention is seductive. Parents allow unacceptable behaviors that instill bad habits, set low expectations and perpetuate a continuing cycle for the game to continue. Adult children create emergency situations and expect parents to rescue them from the emergencies. Instead of learning from the past, they don't see themselves as part of the problem and don't even consider creating a solution themselves. They ask for and expect their parents to rescue them, and the parents do.

This mind game has real consequences as it's played out in real life. The Enable Table puts a strain on each of the participants emotionally, and often, financially. Continuing to rescue without lessons learned, boundaries set or new expectations in place, relationships become toxic and dangerous. Parents, as enablers, feel satisfied in the short run that they are helping. In the long run, they feel hurt, angry, resentful, used and abused as the cycle repeats itself. Adult children, who have framed themselves as victims, feel entitled to relief from the emergency at the effort and expense of their parents. In the long run, these victims/adult children do not have the skills or experience to solve the problems they perpetuated and created. In the game, if the parents decide to fold and end the game, the adult child feels abused and begins to blame with statements like, "You've always done it in the past, and now you won't continue. If you weren't going to do this forever, you should have equipped me with the skills to handle things myself." That's not right, but it's the normal reaction, especially after many years of enabling. The parents must close the table, independently or with professional help. It's like ending a card game. Each party must change behavior. As parents, we must stop taking responsibility for our children's actions. Parents, do you know how wrong it is to hold back our child's maturity in the name of helping? It's toxic. It's as toxic as watering a plant with acid. The toxicity burns away its ability to grow. We're killing our children in the name of helping/love.

In Our Home

Our past mistakes, drama and nonproductive dialogue about their social and emotional immaturity should have been packed away or discarded with their memorabilias as each son exerted his independence. We just remained ready to start where we left off whenever the immature postadolescents returned home. With us having a big house with too many bedrooms our adult sons were very comfortable coming back home. There were plenty of resources available as we were in our maximum earning years and retirement seemed far into the distance. Neither of our three sons demonstrated any antisocial personality disorders. Because we were prepared to assist our sons in conquering any obstacles to become successful, we wanted them to achieve our level of lifestyle. We failed them because they did not develop a realistic sense of financial management and other executive functions, necessary to reach this level.

Frustration is uncomfortable, and discomfort is frustrating. Low frustration tolerance means that, most times, if something was difficult to handle, they became frustrated by the outcomes of their own behavior, and instead of working through the emotions, the challenges and the complex problem-solving to make things better, they quit. Then they would turn to us to fix "it" to make it better and we did. When your child is ADHD and you fix the situation, the child doesn't learn anything. They move on as if nothing happened until the next time that they need the parent(s) to fix "it." That perpetual cycle continues to create problems and more frustration.

Helping is part of a parent's DNA. The more we helped and protected, the more we became addicted to the action. We have experienced with our serial-relationship son, Drew, the excitement of the connection, the stimulation of the actual courtship and the crash of impulsive breakups. Each time, we were there to help for the sake of the grandchildren. At first, it was gratifying to help our son get his footing after a bad relationship. Over time we became addicted to continually rescuing Drew from his own messes, particularly his relationship dilemmas. Behaviors became habits because there was always a safety net. He was looking for a way out and we consistently maintained low expectations.

We believe interrupting the pattern of enabling requires weaning. We say that because once our grandchildren's welfare was at stake, we were committed to keeping them safe, no matter what. Drew manipulated us by using the children, and we know that. We would not have taken care of him all those years if not for them. Weaning, in this case, would have been ensuring they had a stable home in a good school district and an agreement in place to provide a level of financial support for a limited amount of time, instead of using our home as a bed and breakfast where he could just check in and check out at will. Once he moved out and knew there was no coming back, he figured things out for himself. Getting him out of our house sooner would have forced him to be weaned sooner. Had we done that, he would have been able to reflect and plan on his own how to go forward and improve as a man and as a parent.

Controlling makes things worse down the line when your children are on their own. Our oldest son's excuse for his lack of stability is that we enabled him. When he went away to school, he didn't know how to manage his own life. When he became a parent, he didn't know how to make decisions for his children's lives. He said, *"We made things too easy for him, helped him too much."* The excuses don't stop when parents enable. Sure, we know that ADHD weaknesses can lead to educational challenges that affect employment and income potential. The adult child rationalizes rather than analyzes past behaviors. Without hindsight, the past is easily repeated. Complex problem-solving is not necessary if the enablers are consistently operating the safety net. Maturity is arrested when there are limited consequences for classic behaviors. Finally, we realized that our reluctance to set boundaries led to the Enable Table finale. Understanding the role of their inattentive, poor decision-making expectations that our home was a nest with a revolving door meant we needed a contract with our sons to stop the cycle. The agreement would have included: proposed length of stay, contributions to the household, and house rules.

Suggestions for Closing the Enable Table

- Be willing to assess the situation and make suggestions as to how your child can resolve the situation, assuring him you are there for moral support.
- Love, concern, compassion and support for adult children do

not require the same actions as when they were adolescents. When situations arise, be a listening ear and help the adult solve the problem on his or her own.
- If a portion of the problem-solving involves you, the parent(s), and your checkbook, seriously consider if that is the best resolution. If it is decided together that it is necessary, get a promissory note and enforce it.
- A primary goal should be to help build the independent adult; therefore, encouragement, support and acknowledgement of little victories will build esteem and experience for the complex opportunities down the road. Adult children must learn to solve small problems in order to be able to solve larger ones.
- Continuing formal dialogue is essential to maintaining shared expectations. Sit down and seriously talk about what is happening. Treat these interactions as you would any responsible adult-to-adult interaction.
- Lack of financial planning is typically an issue. Be realistic about finances. Take a stand and make a plan to resolve open issues. This is not a one-day conversation and may be difficult to untangle. Effective financial planning takes real effort and tenacity. Do not put yourself as a parent in stressful, dangerous situations that puts your own future at risk. Progress requires effort, and it must be mutually beneficial.

Shutting down Enable Tables requires communication and love, coupled with accountability and boundaries. To open the lines of communication, you may need the help of counselors experienced in these areas.

Falling Through the Ceiling

"Our internal house was a mismatched hodge-podge of impoverished parts, even as the external dwelling looked good to outsiders." – Audrey

Larry was completely afraid of heights and allowed most things around the house to go unfixed. Jay became the fixit man in the family. We moved into an historical house the year Rob graduated from high school. There were many things that needed to be repaired, including a missing pipe in the attic that was needed to divert dripping water from the HVAC unit to a drain. When we saw droplets on the third-floor ceiling, we knew the drain pan needed to be emptied again. Normally Jay would climb up and drain the pan; however, he was no longer living with us and had to be summoned for such repairs. Wanting to be helpful, Rob impulsively took on the task unasked. It did not go well.

> *"Hanging by my midsection, looking down at my mother from the attic to the third floor of our house, I felt like that out-of-control kid who used to write on walls or throw firecrackers into bonfires. How could I have possibly fallen halfway through the ceiling, knocking down plaster and wood onto Mom's head? Jay wasn't even there to dare me to climb up the ceiling ladder from the third floor. He didn't hassle me about being too big to even fit through the ceiling access panel. It was much easier for him, at 5'10" and 150 pounds, to get into the attic. Because I was 6'3" and about 200 pounds, I had no business being up there. Jay's job was always to deftly crawl across the attic beams when necessary. So*

how did I make the decision that resulted in me hanging in that extremely painful position with my sneakers waving above Mom's head? I have no clue. It just seemed like the right thing to do when I made the decision to fix it in the absence of my brother and my father, who was afraid of heights. I was in college; living rent free and was perfectly comfortable with putting off things until later. I guess I thought it would be fun." – Rob

Fortunately, Jay showed up in the nick of time and got Rob down from the hole before he crashed through the ceiling. I felt blessed that once again my child was safe, and at the same time, it was one more atypical day with the Jones Boys. I didn't even bother to ask him why he did it. These types of incidents had been going on for years, and there's never a good explanation. After asking why so many times and it never making sense, you just stop asking and become a fixer—an enabler—to get to the next point. Fixing things is what we learned to do, and it teaches nothing. We had become inoculated against the errors, the mishaps, the poor choices and the bad decisions. Parents will enable until they run out of money, run out of patience or simply give up.

"Rob fell through the ceiling, not because he did not know that beam walking was dangerous, but because he was impulsive. Solving the problem would have taken more effort than trying one more daredevil move." – Audrey

Giving Our Sons a New Start

"Parents continuing to enable adult children simply perpetuate the same behavior. Someone has to decide to stop." – Audrey Jones, after the disaster

Though we told ourselves we had closed our Enable Table, we put a business together in December 2004 so each of our sons would have employment and some foundation for life. It was another disaster in our ADHD life.

Larry found out about a franchise opportunity to provide professional copy and print services in downtown St. Louis. It sounded like a lucrative investment for us and an opportunity for our sons to work, manage and establish their careers while continuing to go to school. Clearly, though unintentionally, we were trying to control our sons' lives. We hadn't yet learned. However, instead of making an informed group decision about the purchase and operation of the franchise, Larry and I charged forward and bought in. As the parents, our plan was that Jay would manage the operation, Drew would market and Rob would work in the store with his brothers.

It was an exciting new adventure for everyone! A feeling of exhilaration and new opportunity overtook our sensibilities, led by ADHD #1, Larry Jones. From day one, our master plan was doomed. The three of them could not agree on their shared or exclusive responsibilities. Also, the business was not nearly as brisk as our projections, not to mention that we opened at the wrong time of year. People didn't know we were open to ship their holiday packages. To top it off, the following week, Larry, who was now working part-time in his private practice and as a medical management consultant for an insurance company, had forgotten to check some details in his noncompete clause and lost his consultancy. The following month, in January, Drew, who had briefly moved in with his pregnant girlfriend, quickly moved out again and into Jay's house. Within 24 hours, he was in the ER with a laceration. Now Drew could not keep his part-time job, was unable to do marketing for the store and was homeless, as his brother had kicked him out for carelessness. He then moved back home with us and was forced to work at the store on crutches as a clerk, unable to do the critical outside marketing. It was a mess. With the store not doing well, I started going into the store to keep the business afloat. Me coming in and attempting to solve the problems was not empowering them to grow; it was enabling them to do only what was comfortable, not what was necessary to maintain and grow the business. Drew and Jay argued about everything. He resented working for his younger brother and refused to shoulder his share of the responsibility.

Meanwhile, Rob, who had been a good employee and did what Jay told him to do, moved to Cincinnati with his future wife and took a job at another store within the same franchise, seeing as he had experience. He built on those skills and became business service manager for a law firm in New York when his wife's career led them to the big city. He's gone on to work in sales and training in the tech industry, and they are doing well on the East Coast.

Back to St. Louis.

In hindsight, we did not make the hard decisions that need to be made when risking large amounts of money. We just gave the boys a business and said, "Go run it." Then when it didn't work well, some of it due to factors beyond our control, the parents attempting to ride in on a white horse to straighten things out was the wrong action.

Drew continued to float in and out, half doing his job at the store. The fact that we were allowing him to live in our home and keep his job, still enabling him, really angered Jay, and rightfully so. Once again, we did not hold Drew accountable for his actions. Drew was now a parent with several children, and the thought of firing him or kicking him out was too much to bear as we considered the fate of our beautiful grandchildren if we did so. That was not the way we should have handled things.

This pattern continued for nearly five years as Jay managed the first and then a second location for the franchise commitment term. In the midst of it all, Jay completed his graphic arts degree, honed his skills and built his résumé. He successfully used his graphic design skills within the store, offering those services to the customers. We started making money and received awards, and yet Jay was becoming more disgruntled with our interference and his brother's slacking. When I got sick in 2008, Jay was left to figure things out on his own, and he had finally had enough. He relocated to Texas in 2010 and immediately took a management position in another franchise store there. He built on those skills, eventually taking a position as manager of media at a university. He lives there with his wife, who is a chef, and is finishing his second degree.

After Jay left, Drew worked at the store sporadically and continued to move in and out of our home. He recognized that he needed to improve himself and found interest in the skin care industry, becoming licensed in the field. He has excelled in sales and management and has worked for a major national brand for several years now. On the home front, he and the kids stayed and took care of me through the crisis time of my illness and until Larry and I downsized into a smaller home.

They Had to Do It Their Way

Larry and I had always thought, *"Boy, if someone had been there to help me, I could have done it so much better, or more quickly."* So that's what we thought we were doing for our boys, helping them. That works in certain circumstances, but not in ours. It translated into enabling their unproductive behaviors and actually stunting their progress, growth and maturity. We did it out of love, yet it still wasn't the right thing to do. When we couldn't stop the cycle, our grown sons stopped, and we adjusted.

"Opening a business for them to operate, I thought, was a part of the American dream. I guess I was forgetting my place as a first-generation–educated Black woman. I was supposed to be home stretching my husband's salary and nurturing my sons to be second-generation–educated Black men. But my parents' sacrifices and determination and Wellesley College convinced me that hard work meant being wife, mother and successful businesswoman, and it meant creating a legacy for my sons." – Audrey

Being the Enabler Turns Deadly

I was a multitasker because I was forced to be, I had so many things to do, and because I felt responsible for nearly everything. I felt like I was *Falling Through the Ceiling* some days just trying to cope. I am admitting this today because what I did was wrong. I want someone else to do right. Let's face it: I was *the Enabler*. Not dealing with the underlying issues but fixing urgent problems in the moment is what I did as my children grew up and my husband worked. They relied on me. I took care of all of them. It all changed one day when I could barely take care of myself. Everyone nearly lost it due to my unexpected illness, which happened as a result of me not taking care of myself.

I had an acute attack of a rare autoimmune disease called autoimmune hepatitis. Autoimmune hepatitis is a disease in which the body's own immune system attacks the liver and causes it to become inflamed. It's as if you had systemic lupus erythematosus, but all the symptoms are concentrated in one area—in my case, the liver. I had been ignoring the fact that I had asthma and had been having annual bouts with pneumonia for nearly six years as a result. When I was 58, the pneumonia hit me again, and I refused to follow through with treatment. When I finally went in to my internist, she gave me some pretty serious antibiotics, and the neurologist had prescribed Gabapentin for the neuropathy, which I was on for several months. Both drugs attack the liver; some people's livers just shut down. Mine did not shut down completely, but my body had an autoimmune response. The effects were that the liver didn't process well, causing all types of gastrointestinal symptoms (diarrhea, vomiting and a lot of pain). The compromised liver stops regulating and allows the buildup of ammonia in the brain. (Normally, the liver gets it out of your body.) Ammonia causes poisoning of your brain and kills cells, causing cognitive deficits; put together, it can become a type of dementia.

My condition forced me into disability in 2008. I could no longer manage a business—because it takes multitasking to do that. I had successfully owned and operated airport concessions and retail locations throughout the region for 24 years while simultaneously managing my husband's medical practice for most of those years and co-parenting our three sons. My short-term memory was almost completely shot. Long-term memory, speech and speech comprehension were all affected. I couldn't even finish a sentence on some of my worst days. When it all collapsed, for a time, I was unable to function without written notes. I missed appointments and even airplanes when I didn't write things down. More than simple notes, I had to create outlines to function, describing what each task was supposed to look like, similar to creating a quilt one little square at a time.

Having a husband and sons who all had some levels of ADHD caused each of them to have their own selective memory did not change their short attention spans and "now, not now" impulses. My illness and recovery caused hell for my family. It reduced and almost eliminated my ability to manage this group of ADHD people who had relied on me to keep things going. They could not believe the 180-degree change they saw in me. *I'm almost ashamed to admit this, but can you imagine that these four men thought I was faking my illness because they relied on me so much?* They felt that I should just get up and manage everything as I had always done. They expected me to wear my cape as *the Enabler*. They thought *they* were going through hell. What about me? Things fell apart as I could barely speak, was continuously falling and couldn't even drive myself. After nearly 40 years of marriage and more than 30 years of motherhood, they didn't know, couldn't relate and frankly didn't care about the hell I was experiencing.

Larry explains:

I really was afraid that Audrey was going to die, and there was no way I could explain that to her. I resorted to being clinical and vague because I was struggling with my own feelings about her illness. The other person who had really loved me (my mother) died and left me when I was 19. I could not go through that pain again. As I have learned through counseling, I never really got over my mother's death. My feeling of being lost caused Audrey to think that I didn't care. I just did not know what to do and my sons were in outright denial that their mother was really sick. Drew came to realize that she was behaving differently when she started sleeping all the time and couldn't remember anything. As he was the only son living in town, he could see her weakness. Like most parents, Audrey would attempt to hide her illness and act like she was feeling much better than she really was when the other two were visiting.

Six months after I got sick, living day to day with an uncertain prognosis, Larry went on the road and took a medical administration position in another state. This choice forwarded his career, but left me behind with a large house to maintain, occupied also with our oldest son and his two children, at the beginning of my rehabilitation. At the time, Drew was in his mid-30s. He felt he was staying to take care of me (doing us a favor), when primarily, he stayed for the convenience of having a safe place to live with his children. He could see it was difficult for me to take care of myself, and he knew that his dad being gone was a result of him not being able to handle seeing me in that condition. Our relationship did evolve as he began to care for my basic needs, use his own resources to care for the children and became committed to taking care of me. Being in our home together, under those conditions, we acted like a loving family and provided safety for us all. Yes, I further enabled Drew because of the grandchildren, but they were ours, we loved them, and they were talented and cute. Plus, Drew was showing growth as he took over my care and the care of his children.

> *"I had devised my own plan where I thought I could save her by taking her out of St. Louis, where she could have a calmer lifestyle, but I neglected to have those discussions with her. By that time, she was beginning to recover and think better as her liver started functioning again. The fog that she had been in for months was starting to clear."* – Larry

To clarify, the town in which Larry was working had a tiny country store, was 20 miles from the closest major chain grocery store and 80 miles away from a city. He had ADHD delusions of grandeur, thinking I would want to and be willing to live in that town where he was "the diversity." As the chief medical officer, he was the only person of color on staff and in the entire community. No thank you. I could not and would not leave St. Louis, where I had excellent medical care, our home and people who looked like me and loved me.

Just when we had moved into a small house for Drew and me and the kids he informed me that they were moving in with another new family. At this point, we stopped enabling him, because at this point, Drew had made his own decision, establishing his own terms for himself and his family but I didn't agree with his choice, afraid it wouldn't work based on the inconsistency of his choices. I renewed my focus on my health and dealing with the short-term absence of my husband. However the reality was that I yearned for a family bond that didn't exist. I didn't want my son to leave. I needed my husband and he wasn't there. I had to acknowledge the hurt and despair I felt, though I loved my husband and sons.

Today, Drew is moving forward with that blended family and his partner is supportive of him. Their long-term familial relationship required him to mature and grow. Our eldest grew from a man-child into full adulthood and became a role model for his sons.

It took time, plenty of therapy and earnest prayer to get through those years. The good news is that my liver is restored; it began regulating again, reducing the toxins in my brain. I have partial restoration of my faculties—not a whole lot, but some. Since I had survived, I came up with some work-arounds to keep going, so things like taking copious notes continue to help me. When it comes to being *the Enabler*, I remind myself that my life, mind and body are on the line—literally as serious as life and death for me—so I handle things differently. In the past few years I've gotten better, thank goodness. Now when my sons call me with a problem, I just say, "No, I don't know the answer, but I'll look it up." (That's a joke! They have learned it means I'm expecting them to figure out things for themselves.) If it's a real problem, I apply the tools/methods I've learned to help them figure out the problem themselves. If I could go back, I certainly would do things differently. However, I did the best I could with the Jones Boys and my husband.

ADHD Affects Everything from Money to Marriage

Throughout our lives, I felt we had been like Rob the day he attempted to balance on the rafters in the ceiling. We were always trying to stop ourselves from Falling Through the Ceiling. We thought we could move from beam to beam, secure in every step; we were actually teeter-tottering on the rafters when we thought we were balancing all the things we had going on. In fact, we were on the brink of falling through the ceiling as we attempted to balance our careers, manage my illness and enable our eldest son.

"Rather than shutting down, we chose to open up and tell our story." – Audrey

Money Matters and Materialism

"Prolonged attempts to fix the unfixable can deepen into destructive patterns that can ensnare the relationship or the entire family structure." – Gina Pera, author of Is It You, Me, or Adult A.D.D.? Stopping the Roller Coaster When Someone You Love Has Attention Deficit Disorder

When Larry was being inventive with limited funds during our courtship, I thought it was attractive. The reality was Larry was resourceful because he didn't have backup resources. Whatever he earned in summers and at college had to cover everything not provided in his scholarship. Submerged in the high-income New England college environment, everything was free or extremely expensive. He learned how to fake it or find a sponsor. By junior year, he even had money for splurging on dating. However, I had never considered what it meant to not have parents covering my school budget. Sure, I had summer jobs during college, but the money went for shopping and leisure travel. When we merged our incomes, dilemmas arose quickly. Throughout the years, we continued to struggle with the way we spent money, as I often felt it was wasted on material possessions heavily influenced by Larry's gift of Inattentive Type ADHD.

The Way We Saw Money Affected Our Values and Our Marriage

Although Larry's mother was proud and refused public assistance, even when she was too ill to work, he started working odd jobs at an early age, even selling potholders door-to-door. It was his uncle who was his financial role model. Uncle Mickey was a childless, heavy-drinking gambler whose standards were new Ford Thunderbirds, fancy clothes and jewelry on a hotel doorman's wages. Uncle Mickey provided Larry with fashionable clothes and misplaced values. I got a glimpse of Mickey's lifestyle when, shortly after our wedding, we visited him in his low-rent apartment with the new Thunderbird out front.

Larry's ADHD only intensified his materialistic expectations. I did not understand the trade-offs on the financial road in front of us. During the courtship, we agreed on over-the-top dreams, but made few financial plans to achieve them. Like most couples in their early 20's, just out of college, we plunged naively into excessive credit card debt, furnishing our townhouse and even purchasing a new car for cash. With my full-time income and Larry's medical school grants, we thought we were secure. We learned a lot through those experiences, especially after our car was wrecked and due to insurance restrictions and our lack of savings, we were unable to get it replaced. Once after our first son was born, Larry forgot all of his clothes and the baby's new layette at the laundromat because of his inattention to the task. Each item had to be replaced, and I insisted on a washer/dryer at the house to avoid future laundromat mishaps. Incidents like these happened quite frequently, and as a result, our financial issues spiraled, creating long-term consequences. We established an unhealthy pattern of spending and simply justified it by adding debt especially as our incomes grew, versus reigning in spending and making better choices.

Soon I was in graduate school, which meant more student loans, while working and being pregnant *again*. It was time for a house, but we had poor credit despite a good income. The affordable houses were limited in the school district where we wanted to settle. When we couldn't come up with the down payment for a modest bungalow, the seller gave us a second mortgage. We had already accepted down payment gifts from the relatives. With our inattention to details, we had bought a house that couldn't pass the local inspection. We hadn't read the fine print, which the seller took advantage of. There was a geyser bubbling right out front, yet we were stuck with two mortgages and lots of water. But by the grace of God, we moved into our first house and somehow made it through.

The next expensive, impulsive choice was a full-time sitter with a *third* baby on the way. Surely my new master's degree in health administration would provide more income than staying home to care for the brood. The bungalow immediately felt too small. Meanwhile, we finally replaced our broken car. Even though I had been raised in a home with indulgent parents, they taught me to plan and save first.. Even when my parents advised against our early extravagances, I never took time to heed them or catch my breath—notice the reckless spending—or to save.

We Didn't Change Our Spending Habits, We Just Worked Harder

His less obvious behaviors prompted Larry to disguise his spending and make choices that put us in financial jeopardy. When we first started out, we were more than flat broke, pinching every dime, wondering how we would make it with our increasing debt and increasing family. When his college and medical school loans kicked in, along with a new baby, it seemed like an unfixable roadblock. But Larry was creative, working full time while also doing a full-time fellowship, there by bringing in two incomes. We used these incomes to repay student loans and fund our household expenses. A sense of entitlement came with each new upgrade, be it cars, housing, accolades in career or financial revenue increases. Funded with credit cards, we started attending "tax-deductible" medical conferences all over the country, staying in expensive hotels with one, two or three of the babies in tow. This spiraled into more expensive events each year until our last family vacation. Larry's impulsive decision-making has always been the most costly as he promotes his career. The lifestyle he envisioned was accommodated by Larry's financially successful medical practice and my business endeavors. As long as there was revenue to pay for the purchases he desired, we kept spending and taught our sons the same thing, vicariously, as they enjoyed the products of our lavishness.

Because we didn't know about and understand how ADHD was affecting our financial decision-making, we usually ended financial discussions (aka arguments) with him shutting down and me compromising my way into another financial loss. With the non-affected person—me—acting as a fixer, I was helping to fund the madness rather than planning how to turn it around. Impulsive purchases and investments decreased our disposable income and savings. Plus, we consistently used short-term debt to cover these mistakes. Several times, we were overwhelmed by credit card debt and taxes, plummeting both our credit ratings.

I knew better, at each of these steps! Yet I began to and continued to cosign with my husband and did not apply what I knew when he made these decisions. When we were newly married and raising our infants, we made one bad decision after another; it didn't even change as we matured. Instead, we kept making more money to meet our financial carelessness. Any time we got to the edge, we made more money; then the kids needed more, so we kept working harder to make more money and fix the finances. We were fortunate to be able to work hard and earn more. However, the pressure of working, earning and compensating for everything contributed to my illness.

Starting in another doctor's office, he quickly moved into a individual practice with me as office manager. I had supported the operation, so Larry barely knew how to use a computer. He came in late, took great time with each patient and counted on me to do the rest. I could never afford to give up my responsibilities of keeping the distracted doctor on track. ADHD behavior negatively affected our bottom line. Starting the workday late meant overtime for the staff. Not billing newborn visits on time lost direct revenue. The practice decisions were his to make and mine to clean up. Money wise, even when running my own business, Larry's perception was, "What's yours is mine and what's mine is mine." That included him managing the home accounts so I was unaware of his sometimes extravagant purchases. After finishing my MBA when Rob was five, I was ready to move on to what I hoped to be a more personally satisfying career. When I left to start my first business, Larry's Pediatrics practice rapidly declined.

In addition to traveling to the medical conferences, there were the lavish vacations that he planned and I agreed to. Often, we went to see or vacation with former classmates and friends to show how well the "poor southern boy" was doing now. In hindsight, they were all probably "fronting" like we were. To keep up these travels while paying private school tuition for three boys meant constantly looking for travel bargains and working even harder to pay for what we couldn't afford.

What We Learned:

- Do better because you know better; even if it requires counseling and mediation.
- A couple must make wise joint financial decisions. It is not enough to keep your money separate.
- Being in financial jeopardy is stressful, particularly when you don't have the same money management experience.
- Marriage includes "what's his is also hers" for all finances, which includes debt.
- An ADHD partner has trouble balancing wants and needs. Do not continue to cosign their erratic or impulsive financial decisions.
- Financial decisions require the best problem-solving abilities of both parties.
- Set short-term as well as long-term goals.
- Financial friction is a leading cause of unhappy and failed marriages.
- We are inextricably tied to our spouses or mates by contracts for borrowing or purchasing.
- As long as you keep going down the same rabbit hole, you will never get ahead.

What We Should Have Done:

- Become financially literate.
- You can't fix your finances by earning more; you have to change your behavior.
- Love is a key motivation for changing behavior for both partners.

- Parenting is the most expensive financial decision in a couple's relationship.
- Openly communicate feelings about finances; stop cosigning on bad financial decisions.
- Jointly find the right level of financial counseling to resolve debts and learn to realistically plan for future expenses.

Love, Friendship, and Marriage

"We ignored the red flags ..." – Audrey

Red flags are indicators that danger is present and can save your life if you take heed to the warning. Too many times we ignored the red flags, and they almost took us, and our children, under.

Married for 45 years, we spent many of those years piecing together our lives and making big decisions without healthy communication and without being on the same page. We had been devoted to loving each other and our three sons, however the way we showed love was nontraditional in many respects. Our unique backgrounds, personalities and issues resided under the surface. For too long we thought we were individuals from different childhood circumstances with common educational experiences and moral values. However we missed important signals that would be detrimental to our family and future.

Larry dismissed his behaviors as his personal idiosyncrasies and so did I. The bottom line is that if we had paid more attention to his behavior and challenges, perhaps seeking outside counsel, the trajectory of our lives would have been different. But, we did not. He went many years being undiagnosed, and here we are. ADHD is the designation used to group inattention and/or impulsive behavior. It has been diagnosed in three generations of our family: Larry, our three sons and our grandchildren. Yes, it is frequently seen in clusters in families, so once a child is diagnosed, look for it in other family members.

Our Truth

- Denial does not change the diagnosis or help the family. Our sons, after their evaluations, recognized the same behaviors in their father. We should have been evaluated along with them.
- Reflecting on our marriage, I should have pushed the stop button instead of waiting for time to resolve the issue. I just kept enabling the same behavior because I felt I couldn't take the time to stop and look for a better way.
- We were generally in a state of crisis resolution with poor communication. Larry completely shut down when faced with shouting and confrontation. I was raised with middle-aged adults who always argued it out. To cope and stay married, I compromised my way into many emotional and financial losses to deal with the way Larry communicates.
- Every child should be raised in a home where the goals are to communicate effectively, learn group problem-solving and control personal behavior. We missed the mark because we were focused on resolving the ADHD crises in our home. Early intervention and positive coping skills are necessary to motivate children to communicate and to reduce the need for emergency resolution.
- For many years our lifestyle was an internal mess. Medication helped Larry replace irritability and impatience with empathy.
- Keeping the marriage or love flame burning requires reaffirming the positives that created the initial attraction to each other including the gifts of ADHD. Couples should spend time away from their children to reassess their relationship. Elaborate plans are not required. This was a necessary but difficult, emotional shift for each of us. With ongoing individual and couple therapy we have found mutual respect, improved communication and empathy for each other.

Braiding the Circle

"We struggled but stayed together, with faith." – Audrey

There is still hope. We are grateful for the anchor of our shared faith, the anchor our leaders and members provided, and the lasting ties of like-minded people who remain so important in our lives. There was a time when we had become slaves to enabling the controlled chaos. After all that God had brought us through we did not study our past behaviors; we just tried to keep up appearances for the next generation. It wasn't working. Our similar values tied us together—trusting in God and recognizing that God had brought us places we hadn't anticipated being. We shared that faith from the beginning and we grew in that together. We were like two vines from well-rooted pots, becoming braided and making one tree at the top together.

Our relationship was not codependent; it was a supportive circle in which we completed each other, which is what a marriage should be. At first, you are unhappy about it not being 50/50, but the longer you are together, it's easier to support each other, becoming a continuous braid of support with one person doing more sometimes and the other taking over at other times. I didn't start out knowing about the ADHD in Larry, but as we lived the journey, I gained greater understanding of my partner, knowing that I was doing more, but being okay with that. When I got sick I was unable to keep up the circle of support. Bam!

The circle broke. Larry had to be the clinician, business manager and family manager. He had to be everything our family needed with our adult sons and grandchildren to parent, and our businesses to operate. My illness triggered Larry back into the adolescent trauma of losing his mother. My diagnosis was possibly terminal, yet he wouldn't face it and certainly wouldn't answer my questions about my prognosis. For his world to be okay, I had to be okay, as far as he was concerned. He couldn't process my poor health and sudden-onset dementia. It was too much for him to deal with. We began having a hard time because I felt so helpless and I felt his responses were not helpful. They were just clinical, not loving, caring or soothing. I needed warm fuzzies from my husband. He needed a reprieve.

In our 37th year of marriage we started working with therapists to address our broken circle. Medication alone gave Larry a greater ability to listen and actually hear what people were saying. It also gave him a new clarity because he didn't have to probe any longer. He understood what people were saying the first time, but then became too direct, and impatient. Counseling helped him to recognize who he was versus how specific ADHD behaviors had made him compensate to survive. Now he could process information and make decisions within his own personality style. With the help of counselors we developed a new relationship based on understanding each other's strengths and abilities. We developed a new system based on the reality of what my current health now allows to do. I didn't bounce back to complete recovery from my illness. I can walk, drive short distances and perform the necessities for myself and him, with assistance. Therefore he has taken on more responsibilities in the circle, which we've redefined together.

We consider ourselves thankful and blessed to have found each other. I think the mistake some people make is not having shared values when they meet and then they try to compensate for it later. That doesn't work. But most of the time those activities are not strong enough to keep you together. It's even more difficult when children and grandchildren are involved. When you add offspring who also have ADHD, matters are further complicated and volatile situations easily explode. Your expectations and values have to be on the same page. You have to find someone to build a life with who shares your beliefs.

Larry Albert Jones has been my friend since shortly after meeting in the spring of 1970. Definitely the sparks of attraction flew from that first night we met at a party. He was my type: smart, confident, handsome and tall. As our whirlwind courtship began, within two weeks, he quickly became my friend and confidant. We fitted together intimately and through the companionship of being only children.

Each of us brought our own "me" focus to the budding relationship. Since he was early in the recovery process from losing his only parent, his mother, at 19, I was even more attracted to his strength to hold it all together.

Even being an extrovert, I felt an astounding fit with this hyperfocused shy guy. I realized that I was probably managing the relationship from the beginning and not recognizing it. Looking back over our story our relationship evolved with me as a helicopter spouse, but loving it. Sure, we had plenty of serious disagreements as we blended. Ignoring our family's opinions to make our own decisions was tough. Larry's grandmother didn't want us to marry because she had other plans for him back in Memphis. My parents thought I should finish graduate school first. Starting then, we knew we had to be in sync to prove that we had made the right decision to marry in 1972 as soon as I graduated from college. However, our honeymoon period with his struggles through medical school meant rocky day-to-day juggling with frequent mishaps caused by his inattentiveness to detail. Through it, we quickly gained trust and never lost it.

I have never been unhappy with my decision to marry. The great joy of our marriage, having Drew, Jay and Rob, offset dealing with Larry's ADHD brain in the early years of their childhoods. It was not smooth, but Larry managed to make the decisions for schools and childcare so that I could complete two graduate programs. We started and grew our businesses together. Our partnership evolved as my parents and his grandmother aged and needed our care and support locally. We were of like mind and never hesitated to do what we believed was best for our family. Moving his grandmother and my parents to St. Louis when we had three children under the age of 10 took both of us out of our managed chaos and added a new level of intensity to our family. We had to be attached at the hip to get through those years. Living on faith in God and trust in one another pulled us through to be thankful for the time we had with our loved ones, who lived into their eighties. In the end, we were both orphans, bound by love and friendship.

> *"In the long run we trusted in our decision to marry, not trying to prove anything to anyone else, and that's the decision that truly matters. I feel that from my heart." – Audrey*

Larry's Advice, Especially for Fathers

"Don't get in the way of progress. Be willing to do everything to make your family whole and healthy, even admitting that you're wrong and need assistance." – Larry

I know pride gets in the way of rational thinking and listening. Also, your concerns as a parent may cause you to lose your objectivity. However, if you have ADHD or your child does, it's important to consider some key things. I've created this straightforward list to assist you.

1. **The earlier ADHD is treated, the better and faster the child can develop self- control and positive behaviors.**

    I compartmentalized my self-diagnosis. I felt I could handle it because I'd been dealing with it myself for so long.

2. **Discuss the teacher's school concerns with the pediatrician.**

    Go to your child's pediatrician to discuss his (her) issues. Have the teacher or school counselor write a letter to the pediatrician explaining how the behaviors impact the child's learning. With documentation from the school, the physician will ask you about the behaviors in the home setting.

3. **Running to the pastor or religious advisor and asking him to pray is not going to cut it.**

    Although seeking spiritual counseling and being active in church life can certainly help the entire family, don't rely on unqualified persons to treat ADHD.

4. **Be more concerned about your child's well-being and success rather than the label.**

    Obtaining a diagnosis should be an affirmation not a label, because it shows you are taking control in improving your child's opportunities for success.

5. **There should be no stigma attached to diagnosis and treatment.**

    Treatment should be a combination of counseling and medication as recommended by your child's professionals including the pediatrician and the psychologist or licensed clinical social worker.

6. **Remember that your primary objective is to do what is best for your child. If you find your adolescent or young adult is on a rollercoaster of relationships, it's not the other person(s).**

    You need to suggest that they talk it over with a professional. It is difficult for any individual to do self-counseling or adequate self-evaluation to address relationship issues. It takes time and a skilled counselor to work with you to help you set goals and boundaries for yourself in an ongoing relationship.

7. **Men are often reluctant to go to counseling.**

    You don't want to admit anything is wrong with you or your child. Mothers have usually gone through the process earlier and have felt it. Men don't usually feel the impact of something like this until much later. Resisting counseling is a defense mechanism: if there is something wrong with my child, I must consider there may be something wrong with me. Admitting that is difficult, particularly with a child who doesn't act out, but it is necessary.

8. **Frequent job changes may suggest impulsivity and deficient coping mechanisms in accepting criticism.**

   Internalization of this feedback is not healthy and may be due to your underlying ADHD traits.

9. **A quick temper that results in an action you'll regret tomorrow is a sign of impulsivity and shows a need for anger management.**

   If you have a short fuse it is best in those situations to show a restrained response or possibly give no response at all. Sometimes it's best to acknowledge the disagreement or the feedback then say, *"Let me think about that,"* or *"Let's talk about this tomorrow / next week,"* rather than erupting.

10. **Those gifted with ADHD often have an easier time showing empathy to strangers.**

    In family situations, they display resistance and anger, but may be open to sharing with strangers. Be aware of this and address it if you notice this behavior in your family dynamic.

Audrey's Advice, Especially for Mothers

"Parenting is never a 50/50 proposition in any family" - Audrey

1. **Being a mother means investing 100% of what you have to meet your children's current challenges and prepare them to live as independent productive adults.**

   The gift of ADHD often complicates a father's role and contributions, thus our family life was always challenging especially assessing resources to assist our sons.

2. **Pause, instead of choosing to "go along to get along"; interrupt the old habit or repeated negative interaction; stop the negative cycle of interactions.**

   If these interventions are not in place, which usually begin as verbal clashes it can escalate into violent actions as children become adolescents. It's hard, but necessary to take time in the moment whenever possible, to begin to address underlying issues, not just the current eruption.

3. **Recognize that you cannot do everything for your family. Welcome support and guidance from others.**

   Create a village of others who are encouraging, helpful, and supportive of you and your child (ren). As the mother, allow your child(ren) to be part of groups outside the family with others who care and support them. Listen carefully to the feedback and suggestions of these supporters because they come from love. Ask for their support. This includes attending teacher conferences and other school related events.

4. **Follow through with testing recommendations from teachers and school counselors and psychologists/testers and accept recommendations of professionals, including trying medication if necessary.**

   A child's evaluations may indicate above average intelligence and other classroom disruptions may simply be caused by the pace of the class. Accelerated and varied class placements and groupings may resolve problems. But an ADHD diagnosis does not equal a high IQ. Communicate openly with your child about every step that's necessary for you and your child(ren) to understand their school problems.

5. **Recognize that whatever the parental relationship, every parent involved with a child must develop consistent strategies that do not conflict or confuse the child.**

   Approximately 50% of U.S. marriages end in divorce. The divorce rate is even higher when one spouse displays adult ADHD behaviors. Although my husband was diagnosed as an adult, we are blessed to not be part of those statistics. But the condition may occur repeatedly in multiple generations as it did in ours.

6. **Accept each of your children as an individual, in signs and symptoms and diagnostic results, and most importantly outcomes.**

   Even though the diagnosis may be ADHD, each child and adolescent develops at his or her own pace and the resulting outcomes may not be the same and the resulting actions of each child may not be the same. Individual Educational Plans (IEPs), treatment and counseling plans and other assessments, must be the basis of planning for each child. It helped our family to find a family counseling service after our first son's diagnosis, and we continued this with the other sons.

7. **Correct your parenting mistakes when they arise, or are pointed out to you.**

   Establish guidelines for homework completion and household chores before the use of phones, video games, computers, autos, etc. Medication does not correct parental permissiveness.

8. **Be a motivated role model for your adolescents including healthy eating and physical activity.**

   A balanced diet is good for every child, adolescent, and adult. Sports participation is often a key to improving school outcomes, especially when participation is linked to classroom performance. Pay attention to the role of extracurricular activities, support rather than direct the teens' decision making to build their skills.

9. **Don't enable adult children with physical, social and financial support. This only extends their childhood and depletes your resources.**

   Begin early to teach your child to allocate limited resources, so that expectations for financial support will not extend beyond reasonable timeframes. As stated in the stories, set physical, social, and psychological limits on your ability to support their decisions.

10. **Request ongoing comprehensive testing of your child on a regular basis if it is not suggested by professionals, but don't allow any system to label your child permanently.**

    Current knowledge about your child's condition and available services are critical. You're your child's advocate in supporting his or her future of thriving with ADHD.

11. Teach your child or adolescent to be "his brother's keeper."

Our sons and grandchildren became volunteers by participating with us in all kinds of service programs. Controlling personal emotions, showing empathy, and communicating with new people were sometimes difficult behaviors for them in these settings, but today, they are all complimented for their ability to be empathic and great communicators.

For Parents: Lessons from Our Lives

"Repetition of the same critical, expensive mistakes plagues adults with ADHD. As my distraction and hyper focus have become more controllable, I am a better parent, and my sons and I are close again. However, I cannot regain for them the time in their lives when I should have been using my experiences with the challenges of ADHD to support them through the maze of ADHD and finding their own success." – Larry

We told these stories for families with children with ADHD as an example of **what not to do**. While there is more guidance for families and affected children than when we were living this experience, it is likely that families today will do what we did if they do not seek help and follow the recommendations of the professionals who interact with their children outside the home. We had the means, but lots of money was wasted fixing the consequences of their actions: wrecked cars, traffic tickets, expensive auto insurance. Although these are the typical things that most teenagers do, for us, it was like six times worse—twice as much as the average teenager times three teenagers. These stories demonstrate what can happen when ADHD runs rampant and goes untreated. As a pediatrician, I fell into the same trap as many of the fathers in my practice, thinking that the boys were just lazy and willfully not completing assignments.

The average person might well see us as spoiled parents, with spoiled kids, until you see the long hours we worked to give them better childhoods than we had. As a father, I wanted them to have the two-parent family I did not. I never wanted them to experience not knowing where their next meal would come from as I had. When my mother became ill and my grandmother stopped working to take care of us, we went on welfare and depended on the kindness of friends and neighbors to eat and get through those difficult times.

Knowing the dangers and expenses of those cars, we should have been stricter about them. I was 23 when I learned to drive and had my first car. We all love our children and want them to enjoy life, hoping they do as well as or even better than us. I wanted my sons to be independent with their own transportation since I did not as a teenager. However, I was shortsighted when it came to managing the boys driving responsibilities and the costs of them. Without accountability and responsibility, we ended up spoiling and coddling them.

What We Learned

Don't sweat the easy stuff. Just do it.

> Spend as much time with your infant as possible. Fathers need to bond with their children, just as much as mothers. If possible, dads as well as moms should take as much time as possible away from work to spend with your new baby. Get to know your baby; the better you know the infant, the more you love them. This will give you memories that you will cherish for a lifetime. Feed the baby; change the dirty diapers. Fathers should participate in everything for the baby except breastfeeding. This is as easy as parenting gets.

Listen to your child(ren).

> Parents always share their opinions on everything, including classes and teachers. What is your child's opinion of his/her teachers? Classmates in school? Continue to listen as they grow. Expect maturity in their answers as they grow; their responses should be more complex.

Teach your children to be respectful to their parents, and remember as parents to be respectful of your children.

> Chastise your child at home or in a private place not in front of their friends or your friends. Then teach them to apologize.

If two or more professionals are telling you that your child has a learning issue or an attention issue, you don't need to wait for number three.

Educators, medical professionals or even sports/activity coaches have insight and experience in these matters, so listen to them. When a child stands out in a negative way it affects everyone in the family.

Don't be afraid to get yourself tested.

ADHD may explain frequent job changes you've had, anger issues you may have had with authority or the sudden outburst that makes you quit your job or get fired.

Don't be afraid of professional counseling for ADHD.

Swallow your pride and go to counseling. Oftentimes, the mothers are on board but the fathers are not. Get on board. You can be a best friend to your spouse, make fatherhood and motherhood easier and make your marriage less complicated and more mutually enjoyable. Trash the macho attitude: It's worth the time if it will help your child(ren) and family, because the impact is family-wide, even if you have only one child with ADHD.

Faith based family counseling works for addressing family conflicts.

Family counseling helped us recognize the pressures that were blocking our lives. As a family unit we never went to any kind of counseling, except with our pastor. During their adolescent years our pastor was particularly good at it because he and his wife were parenting as well. He also had three sons and related well to our situation because of his age and his own family. We were always having pressure-cooker experiences and he taught us to really work through things with love.

- o He helped us to remember that the bottom line was that we love each other and that God was blessing us with opportunities.

- He taught us to not let the pressure of problems or big decisions fracture who we are as a family or as individuals.
- He taught us that wrong thing to say is, *"I love you so much that I'm going to pressure you into doing this or doing that."*
- He taught us that love for one another should be demonstrated through respect, kindness and patience versus control, manipulation, selfishness or complete self-focus.

Finally, getting to the root of the "issue" of whatever may be happening is the key to creating healthy behaviors, focused children, managed expectations and accountability, and laying the foundation for lifelong success.

FINAL THOUGHTS

"From the Winds of Frustration to Stabilization and Resilience"
Audrey and Larry

Our family memoir was written to highlight for parents and professionals the journey that our family has taken to get to stability in our marriage and our sons' lives. These are just some of the stories of our parenting experience raising three African American males. As you have read, it has been a wild roller coaster ride of child rearing. We want your path to be more direct by avoiding our mistakes and finding the right tools to guide your child(ren) successfully through the maze of distractions that accompany ADHD. Hopefully you will share what we have learned about how crucial stabilizing inattention and impulsive behaviors are, in order to unlock each person's gifts. This is an ongoing challenge. We want our perspective in *Falling Through the Ceiling* to be a catalyst for discussion and sharing your story with other families and friends.

As a parent reading our stories, you understand the value of early diagnosis and treatment. Early interventions are extremely effective in focusing on the most appropriate educational and behavioral goals. You have the benefit of regular meetings with the school to keep education and behavior on track. You as the parent are the primary decision-maker and advocate. However, as the child approaches adolescence, he should be included in the decision making process.

We were diligent and resilient in getting our sons through high school and transitioning them to college. Based on our college experiences, we thought that college would offer them their best opportunities to thrive, but it was there that they each hit the proverbial brick wall. These years were our greatest tests as parents. We had been a significant stabilizing force for them, and too often, enablers. Even though they had been taught to focus in order to be successful in school. As the stories reveal, our maturing young men each continued to struggle with inattention, hyperactivity, and impulsivity in college. Only Rob completed his bachelor's degree on his first try.

To stabilize our sons and begin to unlock their adult gifts required many resources, a different set for each one. In others words, preparing for a positive lifestyle after the storms and day-to-day challenges of ADHD required resource kits including:

- Family
- Educational professionals (teachers, counselors, coaches)
- Psychological therapists and counselors
- Physicians
- Medication

When our sons began living independently, they disavowed the need for most of the types of resources we had provided. But as they have matured, they have cobbled together their own teams and villages to keep their positive behavior on track. Fortunately, they have found supportive, loving mates that encourage them and establish ground rules for their relationships.

After 40 years of practicing parenting we see that our most critical responsibilities continue to be:

- Keeping realistic expectations for each child, accounting for how ADHD affects him
- Maintaining a stable, safe home
- Providing positive supervision and learning experiences at every age
- Promoting shared problem solving, not enabling, as they mature

Our measure of success is their ability to have meaningful careers, find loving mates and to use the principles we have outlined in this memoir and other principles to raise their children. Each one has told us their stories of how they use their gifts to overcome disappointments and difficulties on their own. Their measurements of success are based on their individual, focused expectations. They have harnessed tools that complement their capabilities for adult focus and self-discipline. We are proud that Drew, Jay, and Rob continue to solve their problems and resolve lingering issues that allow their gifts to emerge and their lives to thrive.

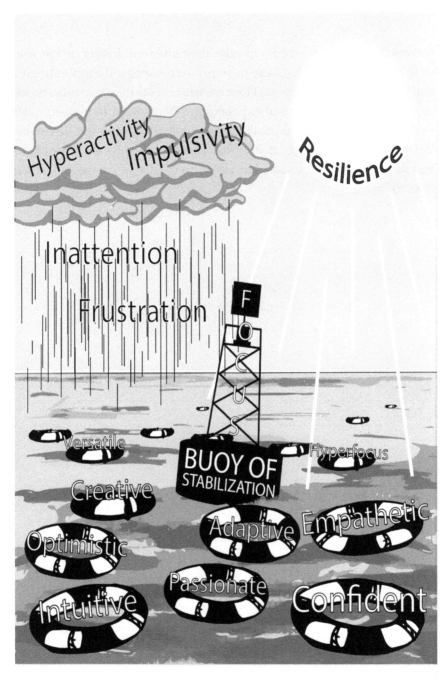

FOCUS - BUOY OF STABILIZATION

FRUSTRATION TO RESILIENCE

The BUOY OF STABIIZATION is the center our image of moving from the clouds of Hyperactivity, Impulsivity, and Inattention toward Resilience.

Falling Through the Ceiling is our advice for stabilizing the effects of ADHD. Resilience is the ability to focus skills and gifts to thrive in adverse circumstances. When negative behaviors are controlled, positive attributes rise to the surface. The positive attributes of the adult ADHD brain are hidden by the failures of past inattention in school, work, and relationships. We witnessed how stabilizing unproductive behaviors over time allowed their natural strengths to the surface.

We see emerging strengths as life preservers that helped our sons regulate their lives, the opposite of falling out of control.

We were struggling to make it and created codependency and unhealthy enabling habits. What we did, and what we didn't do, to help our sons didn't work, many times. The behaviors simply continued and morphed. If we had it to do all over again, we would have done things better and differently. Hopefully our stories will give other parents relief, support, courage and solutions.

- Audrey and Larry Jones, authors, Falling Through the Ceiling

APPENDIX:
What is ADHD?

"ADHD is NOT caused by: poor parenting, falls or head injuries, traumatic life events, digital distractions, video games and television, lack of physical activity, food additives, food allergies, or excess sugar."
Attention Deficit Disorder Association (www.add.org)

Attention-Deficit/Hyperactivity Disorder (ADHD) is a common neurodevelopmental disorder that is usually diagnosed in childhood. However as our story shows, it may be diagnosed at any stage of life. The children's behaviors are consistent problems with paying attention and/or controlling impulsivity which interfere with daily activities. In the long term untreated ADHD affects all types of school performance and maturation. According to CHADD, it affects 17 million people in the U.S. across all types of backgrounds and 60% of adults diagnosed as children have some symptoms as adults.

There are two main types of symptoms: Inattentive Type Presentation and Hyperactive Impulsive Type Presentation. With our sons we experienced problems with both types. When there is more than one affected child in the family it may be difficult to sort out the behaviors as Inattentive or Impulsive. When both types are identified in a person, it is called Combined Presentation. The symptoms changed as they matured, and the challenges became greater for us until each son was tested and diagnosed.

We kept waiting for our kids to outgrow inattentiveness and impulsivity because we knew that all kinds of things cause children to have trouble focusing and behaving in school and at home. But unlike most kids, their ADHD fueled minds continued to cause waves of impulsivity even with professional guidance and medication as they matured.

For the untreated adult similar behaviors persist in workplace and throughout their lifestyle. Work issues are usually the most obvious for some adults with unmanaged symptoms. They also make unexplainable lifestyle decisions; and have costly auto and financial problems. Larry has described the effects on our family of his adult ADHD throughout the memoir.

The Attention Deficit Disorder Association's (ADDA) mission includes focusing on the prevalence of adolescents and adults with ADHD in the criminal justice system. On their website, www.add.org, they estimate that the prevalence is 4 to 8% of adults. But their research estimates that 25 to 40% of inmates in the criminal justice system have ADHD, most are undiagnosed and untreated. Identification and management in childhood could have significantly reduced these sad statistics. Fortunately, ADDA is actively working to improve diagnosis and treatment for inmates in prisons so that they have better outcomes as they leave the prison system.

ADHD is challenging at every age. But diagnosis and treatment can significantly improve life for the child and entire family's experience. The earlier the diagnosis, the sooner improvements are possible. At every age there are opportunities to improve the person's lifestyle by managing behaviors with the correct individualized treatment plan. While the plan may include medication, it always includes behavioral interventions, parent/patient training, and educational support at every age.

APPENDIX :
Advocating for Diagnosis and Treatment

"As the parent, it's up to you to find the resources necessary to nurture and support your child(ren) in growing through ADHD." – Audrey

- Once ADHD symptoms are reported by the school, through appropriate evaluation the primary care physician/ pediatrician should be the first resource consulted beyond the school. Be aware that some schools have a psychologist who may have seen the child prior to contacting the parent. If there is a school report written by the psychologist it should be released to the child's physician for a more meaningful discussion about the child's behavior based on written observations. Also the doctor may use behavioral screening tools to confirm and supplement the findings in the school report. The next step is evaluation by a psychologist for additional testing and counseling to confirm the diagnosis through school or through a private psychologist. This referral can come from the child's physician or from the school.
- If the results of the psychologist's evaluations are consistent with the school's findings, then the physician should discuss counseling and medication. If starting medication is recommended, it requires regular follow-up to review the effects of the medication on the child's behavior; the effect on school performance; and determine if adjustments in the dosage are necessary to obtain optimal results. Multiple studies have

shown that the best results in treating ADHD occur when counseling and medication are used together. Thus, parents should develop an ongoing relationship with the primary care physician and the psychologist as well as the school.

- At this important juncture, it is essential that educators who interact with the child (including the school psychologist), the outside psychologist and the primary care physician, along with the parents, are all operating as a team for the benefit of your child. This can occur only if release forms are signed by the parents to allow these individuals and entities to talk to each other on a regular basis. This input from all of the providers is necessary to accurately develop the individualized educational program (IEP) for the child, which is used to determine necessary accommodations for academic success. This could be more time for tests, homework, etc.
- The Americans for Disabilities Act (ADA) requires an IEP and the availability of testing to complete the IEP through school, public or private. However, getting tested in the school environment can take up to one-half the school year to be completed in large school systems At the beginning of each school year after the diagnosis is confirmed the team shall meet to assess the child's educational progress, review the IEP and update it as your child's behavior performance changes.
- Testing and treatment outside of the school is expensive, unless you have good healthcare insurance. In our 24 years in the Pediatrician's Office we saw Medicaid recipients and professional parents who were steadfast, compliant advocates for their children with ADHD. We worked with all of our parents, who like us, suffered through years of denial about ADHD: "no not our child."
- If you have an urgent need to get an evaluation with no insurance or limited insurance coverage, medical services and psychological services can be obtained at federally qualified health centers (FQHCs) or municipal and county clinics. They usually have both medical and psychological services available.

- You can also refer yourself and your immediate family to an employee assistance program (EAP), if this benefit is available through your employer. An EAP offers employees assistance with personal problems that can impact their physical, mental and emotional well being on the job. This benefit also allows coverage for family members.
- As the child's advocate, be aware that ADHD medications like all medications have side effects that can actually induce or enhance symptoms of other behavioral disorders. These associative disorders include:
    - Oppositional defiant disorder
    - Conduct disorder
    - Anxiety disorder
    - Bipolar disorder
    - Depression
    - Substance abuse
    - Learning disabilities
    - Tourette's Syndrome
- Because of this association, it is imperative that you report any unusual behavior such as frequent crying, agitation, distancing from family and friends to the physician. This might prompt a visit to a psychiatrist for further evaluation for a combination of the disorders above. The psychiatrist might discontinue the medication altogether or change to another medication to treat this behavioral disorder.

One of the scariest things to consider, especially as a person of color, is to have one more negative "label." Further labeling is one of the reasons people refuse treatment for ADHD. They refuse counseling and some refuse both medication and counseling when it's clear something is off. Focus on the well being of the child instead of the label.

Getting to the root of the "issue" of whatever may be happening is the key to creating healthy behaviors, focused children, managed expectations and accountability, laying the foundation for lifelong resilience and success.

Glossary of Terms

ADA Accommodations – Nearly all colleges and universities are subject to the ADA, Section 504, or both. The Americans with Disabilities Act (ADA) provides broad nondiscrimination protection in employment, public services, and public accommodations (including many areas of colleges and universities), for individuals with disabilities. The ADA is enforced by multiple federal agencies, including the Department of Justice, Department of Labor, and the Equal Employment Opportunity Commission. (Higher Education Compliance Alliance; http://www.higheredcompliance.org)

ADD – Attention deficit disorder. Primarily adolescents and young adults who are inattentive but usually reacting slowly, more quietly and cannot control their focus. Added to the DSM in 1980 to replace minimal brain dysfunction. [DSM is the abbreviation for the *Diagnostic and Statistical Manual of Mental Disorders*. It is published by the American Psychiatric Association.]

ADDA – The Attention Deficit Disorder Association (ADDA) is the world's leading adult ADHD organization. We are an international non-profit – **501C** – organization founded over twenty-five years ago to help adults with Attention Deficit/Hyperactivity Disorder (ADHD) lead better lives. (www.add.org)

Adderall – Amphetamine medication; one of the first prescribed for ADHD after Ritalin.

ADHD – Attention deficit hyperactivity disorder. Primarily adolescents and young adults who have trouble paying attention and act impulsively, with high energy. Added to the DSM in 1987 to replace attention deficit disorder.

ADHD and ADD shared characteristics:
- The chemical neurotransmitters in the brain cause different reactions such as impulsivity.
- Both make schoolwork more difficult because of the effect of distractibility on concentration.
- Some characteristics and effects are seen in the majority of diagnosed individuals, but many are hidden.
- Varying effects display for each individual.
- Both disorders run in families, but there is no confirmed DNA marker. However, the characteristics can vary within the same family.
- School performance improves with medications because they can control inattention so that students can improve study habits.
- Both slow maturation from adolescence to adulthood.

ADHD Medication – There are a number of stimulant and non-stimulant medications indicated for the treatment of ADHD.

Amphetamine – Class of stimulant drugs that help students overcome distractions and concentrate.

CHADD – Children and Adults with Attention Deficit Hyperactivity Disorder,. CHADD is a national nonprofit organization that provides education, advocacy and support for individuals with ADHD. CHADD operates the National Resource Center (NRC) on ADHD with the Centers for Disease Control and Prevention (CDC). (www.chadd.org)

Cognitive Enhancers – drugs, supplements, and other substances that improve **cognitive** function, particularly executive function.

Common ADHD behaviors:
- Feeling of constant underachievement and low self-esteem
- Needing intense stimulation to prevent boredom and follow-through on tasks.

- Worrying needlessly; negativity
- Using illegal drugs to calm behavior
- Difficulty managing personal behavior in group settings (i.e., constantly restless, fidgeting, talking; trouble taking turns)

Education Counselor – Licensed professional who guides and mentors adolescents and young adults to develop realistic and feasible plans that match the student's needs and abilities.

Executive Function (EF) – Everyday life management skills:
- Ability to remember and recall facts to make future decisions
- Ability to determine and expend appropriate effort to start and complete tasks
- Ability to control physical reactions to frustration
- Ability to remember and recall multiple facts at the same time, including past events
- Ability to solve complex problems
- Ability to manage time to plan and execute current tasks
- Ability to perceive and plan for future events
- Ability to follow procedures

Individualized Educational Program (IEP) – An educational plan for students with disabilities as defined in federal mandates, including identifying learning problems and specific intervention strategies.

Psychoeducation – an assessment and intervention that targets a student's function within his or her educational setting.

Pschosocial – approach to therapy that looks at individuals in the context of the combined influence that psychological factors and the surrounding social environment have on their physical and mental wellness and their ability to function.

Psychiatrist – Medical doctor who treats mental illness and can also prescribe medication.

Psychologist – Mental health professional who treats clients with counseling and other services but not through prescribing medication.

Psychiatric Social Worker – Licensed professional who assists clients and their families in coping with mental health and related issues in various settings.

Stimulant Medications – the most commonly prescribed medications for ADHD. The stimulant medications indicated to treat ADHD are methylphenidate (Ritalin, Concerta), dexmethylphenidate (Focalin), mixed amphetamine salts (Adderall),[16] dextroamphetamine (Dexedrine), lisdexamfetamine (Vyvanse),[17] and in rare cases methamphetamine (Desoxyn).[18] Controlled-release pharmaceuticals may allow once daily administration of medication in the morning.

Resources

There are many resources by authors who provide detailed treatment guides for ADHD. Because *Falling Through the Ceiling* is simply our family's stories, we did not repeat the experts. This is not a comprehensive list but a compilation of the sources that we used.

Foley, J. M. (2016). *Baxter Turns Down His Buzz*. Magination Press.

Levrini, A., & Prevatt, F. (2012). *Succeeding With Adult ADHD: Daily Strategies to Help You Achieve Your Goals and Manage Your Life*. American Psychological Association.

Nadeau, K. G. (2016). *Learning to Plan and Be Organized: Executive Function Skills for Kids With AD/HD*. Magination Press.

Quinn, P. O., & Stern, J. M. (2012). *Putting on the Brakes: Understanding and Taking Control of Your ADD or ADHD*. Magination Press.

Quinn, P. O. (2012). *AD/HD and the College Student: The Everything Guide to Your Most Urgent Questions*. Magination Press.

Quinn, P. O., & Maitland, T. E. L. (2011). *On Your Own: A College Readiness Guide for Teens With ADHD/LD*. Magination Press.

Vaccaro, P. (2018). Designs On Time. Retrieved from http://www.designsontime.com/

References

ADDA, & CHADD. (2017). *2017 International Conference on ADHD: Connect & Recharge* [Conference Guide]. Atlanta, GA: *n.p.*

(2017, May 31). *Attention-Deficit / Hyperactivity Disorder (ADHD)*. Retrieved from https://www.cdc.gov/ncbddd/adhd/facts.html

(2017). *Attention: Living Well With ADHD.* 24(1).

Bazelon, E. (2016, June). Pulling Strings. *The New York Times Magazine.*

Bottke, A. (2008). *Setting Boundaries with Your Adult Children: Six Steps to Hope and Healing for Struggling Parents.* Eugene, OR: Harvest House.

Comer, J. P., & Poussaint, A. F. (1992). *Raising Black Children: Two Leading Psychiatrists Confront the Educational, Social, and Emotional Problems Facing Black Children.* New York: Plume.

Dawson, P., & Guare, R. (2010). *Executive Skills in Children and Adolescents: A Practical Guide to Assessment and Intervention. 2nd ed.* New York, NY: The Guilford Press.

Dendy, C.A.Z. (2006). *Teenagers with ADD and ADHD: A Guide for Parents and Professionals. 2nd ed.* Bethesda, MD: Woodbine House.

Dendy, C.A.Z., & Zeigler, A. (2007). *A Bird's-Eye View of Life with ADD and ADHD: Advice from Young Survivors.* Cedar Bluff, AL: Cherish the Children.

Graham, B., & Pipher, M. (2010). *Eye of My Heart: 27 Writers Reveal the Hidden Pleasures and Perils of Being a Grandmother.* New York: Harper.

Hallowell, E. M., & Jensen, P. S. (2010). *Superparenting for ADD: An Innovative Approach to Raising Your Distracted Child.* New York: Ballantine Books.

Hallowell, E. M., & Ratey, J. J. (1994). *Answers to Distraction.* New York: Pantheon Books.

Hallowell, E. M., & Ratey, J. J. (1994). *Driven to Distraction: Recognizing and Coping with Attention Deficit Disorder from Childhood Through Adulthood.* New York: Simon and Schuster.

Hallowell, E. M., & Ratey, J. J. (2005). *Delivered from Distraction: Getting the Most out of Life with Attention Deficit Disorder.* New York: Ballantine Books.

Honos-Webb, L. (2008). *The Gift of Adult ADD: How to Transform Your Challenges & Build on Your Strengths.* Oakland, CA: New Harbinger Publications.

Holden, K., et al. (2014). Toward Culturally Centered Integrative Care for Addressing Mental Health Disparities Among Ethnic Minorities. *American Psychological Association, 11*(4), pp. 357-68.

Nadeau, K. G. (1997). *ADD in the Workplace: Choices, Changes, and Challenges.* Milton Park, U.K.: Taylor & Francis.

Patterson, J. (2012). *Middle School: Get Me Out of Here!* New York: Little, Brown and Company.

Pera, G. (2008). *Is It You, Me, or Adult A.D.D.? Stopping the Roller Coaster When Someone You Love Has Attention Deficit Disorder.* San Mateo, CA: 1201 Alarm Press.

Perrine, S. (2016, December). The Bank of Mom and Dad. *AARP, The Magazine.*

Schwarz, A. (2016). *ADHD Nation.* New York: Simon & Schuster.

Shapiro, S., & White, C. (2014). *Mindful Discipline: A Loving Approach to setting Limits & Raising an Emotionally Intelligent Child.* Oakland, CA: New Harbinger Publications, Inc.

Snyder, J. M. (2001). *AD/HD & Driving: A Guide for Parents of Teens with AD/HD.* Whitefish Consultants.

Surman, C., Bilkey, T., & Weintraub K. (2014). *Fast Minds: How to Thrive if You Have ADHD (Or Think You Might).* New York: Berkley.

CPSIA information can be obtained
at www.ICGtesting.com
Printed in the USA
FFHW011523041118
49180433-53393FF